CONCEIVING PERSONS

LONDON SCHOOL OF ECONOMICS MONOGRAPHS ON SOCIAL ANTHROPOLOGY

Managing Editor: Charles Stafford

The Monographs on Social Anthropology were established in 1940 and aim to publish results of modern anthropological research of primary interest to specialists.

The continuation of the series was made possible by a grant in aid from the Wenner-Gren Foundation for Anthropological Research, and more recently by a further grant from the Governors of the London School of Economics and Political Science. Income from sales is returned to a revolving fund to assist further publications.

The Monographs are under the direction of an Editorial Board associated with the Department of Anthropology of the London School of Economics and Political Science.

CONCEIVING PERSONS

ETHNOGRAPHIES OF PROCREATION, FERTILITY AND GROWTH

PETER LOIZOS AND PATRICK HEADY

LONDON SCHOOL OF ECONOMICS MONOGRAPHS ON SOCIAL ANTHROPOLOGY

Volume 68

THE ATHLONE PRESS
London and New Brunswick, N.J.

First published 1999 by
THE ATHLONE PRESS
1 Park Drive, London NW11 7SG
and New Brunswick, New Jersey

British Library Cataloguing in Publication Data
A catalogue record for this book is available from the British Library

ISBN 0 485 19568 2

Library of Congress Cataloging-in-Publication Data

Conceiving persons: ethnographies of procreation, fertility, and growth / edited by Peter Loizos and Patrick Heady.
p. cm. – (London School of Economics. Monographs on social anthropology; no. 68)
Includes bibliographical references.
ISBN 0-485-19568-2 (alk. paper)
1. Human reproduction. 2. Fertility, Human. 3. Body, Human--Symbolic aspects. 4. Sex role. 5. Symbolism in sex. I. Loizos, Peter, 1937– . II. Heady, Patrick. III. Series: Monographs on social anthropology: no. 68.
GN235.C65 1999
304.6′.32–dc21 99-14803
CIP

Distributed in the United States, Canada and South America by
Transaction Publishers
390 Campus Drive
Somerset, New Jersey 08873

Typeset by Acorn Bookwork, Salisbury, Wilts.
Printed and bound in Great Britain by Bookcraft (Bath) Ltd

CONTENTS

CONTRIBUTORS

Dr Ildiko Bellér-Hann trained at the Universities of Budapest and Cambridge and is Research Fellow at the University of Kent at Canterbury. She has long-term research interests in Turkey and Inner Asia.

Dr Andrew Canessa teaches at the University of Essex.

Sini Cedercreutz is completing a PhD in Anthropology at the London School of Economics.

Dr Maia Green teaches at the University of Manchester.

Dr Patrick Heady works at the office of National Statistics.

Professor Peter Loizos teaches at the London School of Economics.

Hania Sholkamy is a consulting associate of the Population Council at the regional office for west Asia and north Africa and a member of the regional Reproductive Health Working Group working on issues related to women's health and to medicine.

Dr Theodore Paradellis teaches at the University of the Aegean.

Julia Stonehouse is an independent writer and researcher.

Ilka Thiessen teaches at the University of Manitoba.

Dr Philip Thomas is a Research Fellow at University College, London.

CHAPTER 1

INTRODUCTION

PETER LOIZOS AND PATRICK HEADY

The essays in this volume are concerned with human fertility in a wide range of mainly contemporary societies. Though some of the societies discussed have been affected by scientific medicine and western ideas about family life, in all of them different local traditions are still strong (or were at the time to which the paper refers). The final chapter discusses the impact of similar traditions on the emergence of scientific embryology itself. The papers are concerned with practices preceding and following conception and birth, and with the ritual processes which contribute to the formation of boys and girls, and fertile men and women.

Collectively speaking, the contributions do not pursue any single theoretical line – though individual authors certainly do. The purpose of this volume is different: to bring contemporary ethnographic data to bear on one of the oldest of anthropology's concerns. We hope that this combination of field sites and theoretical interests will give readers a better idea than any single-focused work could do of the range of issues raised by this perhaps surprisingly complex topic. We hope also that these accounts will stimulate colleagues to speculate afresh on possible new connections between apparently well-known facts – and perhaps to produce new insights based on the societies where they have carried out, or are about to start, fieldwork.

In this introduction we will briefly review some of the most prominent earlier contributions to the literature, and show how they set the context for the papers presented here.

EARLY CONTRIBUTIONS

Questions about procreation have been important to social anthropology since its inception. Indeed, anthropologists' early findings on this topic had great shock value in the late nineteenth and early twentieth centuries. Morgan's (1870) discovery of 'classificatory' kinship terminologies – which make no distinction between an individual's fathers and their fathers' brothers, or between their mothers and their mothers' sisters – seemed to show that group marriage might once have been widely practised. Contemporary reports that some exotic peoples did not even know of the male contribution to procreation made the image of primitive promiscuity seem even more believable. Less luridly, but more subversively and cogently, Morgan argued that the conjugal family of the modern West was not a naturally given form but rather an institutional correlate of a system of private property. This provided Engels (1941) with what he believed – probably rightly – was scientific backing for the radical critique of modern political, economic and family life which had already been set out in the *Communist Manifesto* (Marx and Engels 1848).

But if differences between western and exotic societies could appear subversive, so too could similarities. In *The Golden Bough*, Frazer (1890) produced a vast catalogue of religious beliefs concerning human and vegetable fertility and the link between death and regeneration, which suggested that the central symbols and beliefs of Christianity closely paralleled indigenous beliefs throughout the world. He hardly needed to point out the implications explicitly. All his readers would have agreed that these exotic beliefs were no more than primitive superstitions and, if so, what was Christianity?

The first thorough ethnography of procreation was produced by Malinowski (1932). Though he adopted the analyses of neither Morgan nor Frazer, he was dealing with a society with the features they had emphasized – classificatory kinship terminology, and belief in a cycle of death and regeneration – and had a great influence on the way these topics were treated in academic anthropology. His detailed discussion of Trobriand practices and beliefs was forthright about details of human sexuality, including the belief that women were impregnated not by their husbands but by matrilineal clan spirits. These views were so far from European (or Chinese) beliefs that Trobriand procreation has been a staple of introductory anthropology courses ever since. His account is also significant because it raised three of the issues which have subsequently dominated the anthropology of procreation.

The first of these is the apparent parallelism between ideas about social relationships and ideas about reproductive physiology. In a section on 'the principle of mother right' at the start of the book, Malinowski states

> We find in the Trobriands a matrilineal society, in which descent, kinship, and every social relationship are legally reckoned through the mother only, and in which women have a considerable share in tribal life, even to the taking of a leading part in economic, ceremonial, and magical activities – a fact which very deeply influences all the customs of erotic life as well as the institution of marriage....
>
> The idea that it is solely and exclusively the mother who builds up the child's body, the man in no way contributing to its formation, is the most important factor in the legal system of the Trobrianders. Their views on the process of procreation, coupled with certain mythological and animistic beliefs, affirm, without doubt or reserve, that the child is of the same substance as its mother, and that between the father and the child there is no bond of physical union whatever. (Malinowski 1932:2–3)

The second point, which has already emerged, is the importance of spiritual intervention in human procreation. In the Trobriands this takes the form of a doctrine of reincarnation. The dead go to a subterreanean realm called Tuma where, after existing for a while as adults, they eventually become small spirit children, each of whom 'finds its way back to the Trobriands and into the womb of some woman, but always of a woman who belongs to the same clan and sub-clan as the spirit child itself' (Malinowski 1932:146).

The final issue is the question of how thoroughly procreation dogmas are actually believed. Malinowski's view was clear. Having noted some divergent views on points of detail he goes on to say:

> But that all spirits have ultimately to end their life in Tuma and turn into unborn infants; that every child born in this world has first come into existence (*ibubuli*) in Tuma through the metamorphosis of a spirit; that the only reason and real cause of every birth is spirit activity, are

> facts known to everbody and firmly believed by all. (Malinowski 1932: 146)

Later many other authors engaged in arguments about how far the ignorance or denial of paternal agency in conception was to be believed. Leach (1966) tried to save tribal societies from the charge of 'ignorance' by asserting that their observations of animal reproduction would have left them in no doubt about 'the facts of life'. He castigated some of his colleagues for credulity in accepting the 'ignorance of paternity' argument, and implied a kind of racism. More constructively, he introduced the idea of ideological dogmas into kinship analysis, thus anticipating Bourdieu's (1977) distinction between official and practical kinship discourses. Leach argued that all social systems promote 'official versions' of the ideological beliefs they live by, and that these statements are of a different status from those matters believed on the basis of direct observation. Soon after Leach started making these arguments, other anthropologists came to the view that informant descriptions of unilineal descent as the core organizing principle of their societies were also an official dogma, rather than a comprehensive account of more complex realities (e.g. Peters 1967).

In one element of his argument, however, Leach failed to convince: he reasoned that humans, being good observers of animal reproduction, could everywhere compare their animal-based observations to problems of human reproduction, and draw appropriate analogies. This was a doubtful assumption for two reasons: first, because in many societies humans do not commonly think of themselves as being closely related to animals (Sahlins 1976; Tonkinson 1978), and may be thought of as radically dissociated from them. Second. the very facts of animal reproduction are often complex and obscure, giving rise to imaginative local classification and analysis. Some of the earliest examples of 'ignorance of human paternity' ethnography had been reported in Australia. The reproductive behaviour of some Australian animals may diverge greatly both from animal reproduction in other continents, and also from human reproduction. There is no human analogy to the way in which baby kangaroos and other marsupials are reared up in pouches, and the reproductive physiology of marsupials differs strikingly from that of placental mammals, human and non-human alike (McKnight 1975).

PARALLELS BETWEEN SOCIAL RELATIONSHIPS AND IDEAS ABOUT BIOLOGICAL REPRODUCTION

Among the social relationships that appear to be paralleled by local ideas of procreative physiology, most theoretical attention has been focused on those connected with kinship.

Kinship can be thought of in terms of moral obligations and rights. Some of the most important proceed downward from parent to child and, subsequently, upward from child to parent. Who must feed whom? Who has a right to whose labour? Who inherits what from whom? Who must care for whom in old age, and who must observe funeral rites at whose death? There may also be – usually are – moral obligations to more distant kin, for economic, political, ritual or military support. And there is always an obligation to avoid sexual relations and marriage with certain – culturally very variable – categories of kin.

In most societies there is an expectation that those exercising these rights and obligations will usually be physiologically connected (Barnard 1994:792). In many societies, connectedness is derived in the first place from a doctrine of the transfer of substances from parent to child, and/or the idea that the child is made up from such parental substances. However, the nature of the connection between biology ideas and social institutions is highly controversial.

This controversy arises at least partly because the distinction of biology on the one hand and culture and society on the other has been fundamental to the way that anthropologists, and social scientists in general, have defined our discipline. If we study social and cultural facts, any attempt to reduce them to biology appears to take away our subject matter. (Of course, assertions by anthropologists that kinship is *purely* cultural pose a similar threat to behavioural biologists – and this kind of professional opposition undermines the intellectual quality of both. Ingold (1994) attempts to explore ways in which the two intellectual communities might complement rather than confront each other.)

While it is common ground among anthropologists that kinship institutions and procreative beliefs cannot be *reduced* to biology, many anthropologists have assumed that all cultures will formulate kinship in terms of biological relatedness – so that cultural ideas of reproductive biology must necessarily vary in a way that corresponds to differing systems of kinship institutions. A common form of this assumption is the idea that, although particular notions of how substance is shared and transmitted are as much a cultural construction as the kinship system itself, the basic equation between common substance and kinship is a cultural universal.

This assumption is challenged by Philip Thomas's paper in this volume. He traces the discussion of shared substance back to David Schneider (1984), who identified it as one of two core elements of American kinship. Schneider's earlier work had been on the island of Yap, and he had been careful to state in his reanalysis that the Yapese did not have a 'shared substance' concept of their relatedness. The Temanambondro of Madagascar resemble the Yapese in this. Thomas is concerned that 'substance' is currently used by anthropologists to cover a variety of things, the 'blood' of a descent line, semen, a woman's blood believed to mix with semen in the womb, breast milk, and foods eaten by a set of people sitting together. He suggests that a term used so freely is in danger of lacking explanatory power, and cautions that it is sometimes unclear whether the terms named 'substance' by the ethnographers refer to any distinct concept used by their informants. (The Bimin-Kuskusmin, for example, have two distinct words for menstrual blood and non-menstrual blood and to elide this difference by the analytic term 'substance' surely misses a significant distinction (Poole 1981). Thomas is particularly interesting on the Bara, who are organized ideally into corporate patrilineal groups, think that semen is responsible for conception, but do not give it the same strongly connective biological link to a foetus as the mother enjoys.

'Shared substance, then, is not the basis of Bara "kin groups"' Thomas infers. He does, however, allow that substance is a term 'not without its merits' and most of the contributors to this volume have found uses for it. We would also note that impressive analyses have been based upon it elsewhere (e.g. Daniel 1984; LiPuma 1988, chs 2 and 3).

Since about 1970 feminist anthropologists have been attempting to reanalyse social institutions from the perspective of gender relationships. There is a particularly close connection between the topics of gender relations and kinship, so much so that it is now usual to think of the study of kinship and gender relations as a single subject. In this new intellectual climate it was natural to ask whether culturally defined notions of biology might be as relevant to gender relationships as they are to other aspects of the kinship system.

In 1986 Leela Dube and Carol Delaney independently of each other wrote important articles on the wider gender implications of procreation ideas, and attempted to link them to wider patterns of kinship organization and to major religions. Common to both was the suggestion that in societies which favoured men over women in land ownership, and placed emphasis on patrilineal kinship groups, there was also a male-biased procreation doctrine, expressed in terms appropriate to the production regimes of agriculture. The male contribution of 'seed' to conception was the primary determinant factor, which pushed into mere second place the uterine creativity of the mother. She was only a nutrient medium, like a field.

In chapter 6, Ildiko Bellér-Hann pursues this idea with a comparative analysis of two rural Muslim societies – the Lazi of northeastern Turkey and the Uighurs of northwestern China. Her material on the Lazi confirms this aspect of Delaney's thesis, though – appropriately for a community that practises mountain agriculture – the receptive medium used as an analogy for women's reproductive role was the back-basket rather than the ploughed land. However, among the Uighur the ideology of male supremacy rests on their economic rather than their physiological contribution, suggesting (analogously to Thomas's argument in the case of kinship) that physiological beliefs are not a necessary component of gender ideologies.

So far we have looked at beliefs that trace a connection *from* physical reproduction *to* social relationships. But the connection can be traced in the other direction as well. One of the most common forms of this is the idea that an environment of ill will can damage the physical well-being of mothers and young children. This belief is reported in this volume by Sini Cedercreutz in Indonesia, Ilka Thiessen in Macedonia, Patrick Heady in north Italy and Andrew Canessa in the Andes. Canessa in particular brings out an interesting implication: that the physical well-being of the child depends not only on the parental contributions (however these are understood) but also on the social state of the community as a whole. In Pocobaya discussions and representations of reproductive activities link them as far as possible to religious festivals in which a state of general good will is officially guaranteed.

The notion that physical reality can reflect social developments, as well as the other way round, is consistent with an important emphasis in recent writing about the development of the person, which stresses open-ended social processes, rather than the production of a person 'completed' by the act of birth (Carsten 1992). In contemporary Europe many of us currently think of the cutting of the umbilical cord and the infant's first cry as an existential 'arrival' of a miniature person, dependent but a person nevertheless. There is disagreement on this: 'pro-life' anti-abortionists want to log consciousness and infant personhood much earlier – within the first moments of conception – and regard the moment of exit from the mother's body as of no particular significance; for them, it seems, personhood simply started earlier. But both pro-choice and pro-life Europeans agree that a one-day-old baby is human, a person, and endowed with rights: once the baby is separated from the mother, neither group would accept infanticide of a healthy neonate as legitimate. Their next disagreement might come over the right to life of a severely handicapped infant, and could focus upon the burden of responsibility for an infant if the birth mother is unwilling to nurture it.

But as Strathern (1988) and in this volume Canessa and Cedercreutz insist, the identity of a person can start later too, and may be thought to continue to be modified throughout life, and this is made more complex when the living, breathing person awaits the attachment of a soul to the body. If an interest in process first entered anthropology originally in the Fortesian concept of the domestic group's development, the current concern works at a lower level of abstraction than the aggregate household, aimed at the social transactions needed both to nurture and to organize social placement. In societies where adoption is favoured, (Goody 1982), social placement is contingent, not settled by the fact of birth as membership in a lineage or clan. Cedercreutz's Sulawesi material in chapter 5 draws attention to this issue. Does this mean that the new emphasis on personhood-as-process reflects the identification of regional thoughts and practices common to Malaysia, Indonesia and Melanesia, or is it a more general theoretical shift, which might yield insight into any society, as the comparative material from Europe and the Andes might suggest?

SYMBOLISM, NATURE AND DIVINITY

We now turn to the second theme raised by Malinowski's work: that of symbolism and religious belief. Though this may seem quite a step from the solid ground of social relationships and biological understanding, the transition is less abrupt than might appear. Consider, for instance, what is actually implied by a statement that two relatives share some form of common substance – for instance, the same blood. Before the advent of modern medicine, no one could check this statement: despite the belief that people had different blood, linking each individual with some people but not others, in fact everybody's blood looked the same. Though other socially stressed substances, such as flesh and bones, do observably differ between individuals, it is doubtful whether the biological dogmas refer to these differences. Thus, someone who assures an anthropologist that both sons and daughters inherit their bones from their father alone cannot possibly mean that the bone *structures* of both sons and daughters resemble their father more than their mother. In any case, so far as we know, ethnographic reports of doctrines of the inheritance of flesh and bones never report local attempts to verify the beliefs. It is clear that these biological dogmas have little, if anything, to do with practical understandings of reproductive processes. They are themselves an aspect of the symbolic repertoire which can be used to place procreative processes within the system of social relationships.

In fact shared substance is only one of a variety of things that can be used as metaphors for procreation. Tempting as it may be to fix on a single 'dominant' metaphor, most of the papers in this volume show or imply several sets of metaphors co-existing in a single society. In chapter 10 Theodore Paradellis (examining nineteenth-century folkloric sources as a proxy for modern ethnography) describes the elaboration of three distinct metaphors – cultivating, bread-making and weaving – in rural Greece. Some of the elaborations of these metaphors seem almost playful, but that should not lead us to underestimate either their pervasiveness or their potential importance. Almost every paper in this volume reports some socially recognized parallelism or connection between human reproduction and plant growth: the placenta may be buried in family or village land, or under a suitable tree (Cedercreutz, Canessa, Green). Connections may be drawn between the natural forces of plant and human reproduction.

It is interesting too that these metaphors often involve important productive activities. The three metaphors discussed by Paradellis arguably involve the most important productive activities of each sex. We have already noted the use of metaphors of plough and soil, and back-baskets to draw a connection between production and reproduction in agricultural societies. Even the relationship between sailors and their boats can be metaphorically sexualized, as Cedercreutz reports for Sulawesi. The implications of all this metaphor and symbolism are, as yet, under-theorized, but they are consistent with a strand of anthropological thought going back as far as Mauss which argues that schemes of social relationships include things as well as people – and that relations with things and people are often understood in strikingly similar ways.

Another feature of the symbolism reported by several contributors to this volume is the stress on energy. The connection between human reproductive power and the power of rain and of the sun and moon – stressed in this volume by Canessa and Heady – confirms the findings of earlier authors who have recorded ideas relating human fertility to the lunar cycle (du Boulay 1991; Pina-Cabral 1986) and the dew (Barth 1967). But power, or energy, are seen as important even when only human reproduction is at issue. Cedercreutz's account of ideas about bodily heat in Sulawesi, and Thiessen's description in chapter 9 of Macedonian ideas about the reproductive consequences of the strength of each sexual partner, are cases in point. Is it possible that the implicit dynamism of these ideas about energy, or 'life force', has an affinity with the notions of personhood as process – rather than fixed substance – discussed above?

Ideas of energy and life force are central to many – possibly all – cosmological schemes, and hence to the symbolic legitimation of social and political power. Frazer (1890) and Hocart (1927) provided early and influential accounts of the way power-holders were represented as vessels channelling the forces of divine and natural fertility, but more recent versions have drawn at least as much on the insights of Lévi-Strauss (1969). The first of these was his view – no less influential for being hotly contested since – that all societies draw a distinction between the creative forces of nature and the ordering power of culture.

The social implications of this implied mistrust of nature were first taken up by Ortner (1972) in her theory that male power was legitimated by an implicit identification of masculinity with culture and femininity with nature. Bloch and Parry (1982) drew on a similar insight to rework the Frazerian view of divine authority as a means of channelling natural fertility. Instead, they argue that the symbolism of death and rebirth contrasts with the corruptibility of the natural processes associated with female fertility, replacing it with the image of an incorruptible, timeless, divine fertility under the politico-religious control of old men. They pointed out that in ritual practices, death and reproduction were often inextricably linked, and that 'almost everywhere religious thought consistently denies the irreversible and terminal nature of death by proclaiming it a new beginning. Conception and birth are the most striking and obvious symbols available for asserting such a dogma' (Bloch and Parry 1982:9). Their essay stressed the ambiguity of biological reproduction as a symbol, and pointed to common linkages of sexuality, and particularly female sexuality, to death symbolism. In many rituals they could identify a conceptual de-linking of group reproduction, a 'social' project in the hands of (often male) senior persons, from the 'messiness' and anarchic spontaneity of merely biological, 'wild', and often female sexuality. In ritual symbolism, the social was often found to dominate and marginalize the biological.

On the whole, the essays in this volume pay little attention to the cyclic connections between death and birth, and the material that is reported does not fit very neatly into Bloch and Parry's scheme. It is impossible to read these ethnographies without being convinced that all these societies value natural fertility as a good in its own right – and that this conviction is embodied in symbolism as well as in practical life. Canessa, the only author to describe a full cosmological cycle, reports that the dead are identifed with the beneficent powers of *mother* earth. Though the Greek symbolism described by Paradellis clearly does denigrate sexual fertility, it is far from denigrating natural fertility as a whole. Although this does provide some support for Bloch and Parry, it is not enough to sustain their attempt to stand Frazer's theory on its head. Indeed, Canessa's account of the political implication of Pocobayan ideas about fertility fits in with a renewed interest in the role of procreative and fertility symbolism in modern ideologies of nationalism (Banal and Verdery 1995). It is a detailed working-out of themes which the literature on European nationalism tends to treat in a much less systematic way.

Three contributors to this volume took as their starting point Delaney's analysis in *The Seed and the Soil* (1991), which we have already discussed in the context of parallelisms between social relationships and biological doctrines. But it can also be seen as an attempt to synthesize these ideas with Ortner's (1972) extension of Lévi-Strauss, and with another key Lévi-Straussian insight: the notion of structural parallels between different spheres of social life. These themes are bound together in Delaney's account of a Turkish village in which life was organized round a single dominant metaphor of male generative creativity, which she linked with the idea of monotheism – arguing that the Islamic religion supports the idea of an all-powerful creator god, and that men see their own role in giving patrilineal semen, and in tilling the soil, as equally the decisive sources of creativity and legitimate control.

The papers in the present volume react to Delaney's thesis with some scepticism. Ildiko Bellér-Hann and Hania Sholkamy take issue with her account of Islamic practices and beliefs, challenging the idea that they are monolithic. Bellér-Hann, as we have seen, describes two Islamic societies with markedly different systems of kinship and procreation symbolism and suggests that the symbolism of production compensates for, rather than simply reinforces, the symbolism of reproduction. In chapter 7 Sholkamy points to the existence of several distinct traditions of both learned and popular Islamic thought and shows that Islamic scholars have long held a duogenetic version of physical conception. (It might even be called trigenetic if the later, and distinct, act by which God provides the foetus with a soul is taken into account.) Heady tests Delaney's theory in the context of another religious system, Roman Catholicism, as experienced by villagers in northern Italy. Although his findings lend some support to Delaney's ideas about the interconnection of different social spheres, the parallelism between monotheism and a masculine monopoly of legitimate fertility is not supported. This conclusion is consistent with some problems which Dube's analysis of Indian procreation metaphors implicitly raises for Delaney's approach. Delaney is concerned to link the seed-and-soil metaphor to patriarchal monotheism. But Hinduism, the type case of a polytheistic religion, also sustains both seed-and-soil metaphors, *and* strong patriarchy. If seed-and-soil metaphors are compatible with two such contrasting religious systems as Hinduism and Islam, logically the metaphors cannot play a decisive role in either.

THE QUESTION OF CONSISTENCY AND BELIEF

This brings us to the third issue implicitly raised by Malinowski's Trobriand ethnography – the question of belief. In the past couple of decades, anthropologists have become much more cautious than they once were of attributing unified belief systems to entire populations. In the place of an implicit doctrine of social determinism, more emphasis is now placed on individuals' autonomous efforts to understand and manipulate the world in their own interests. Though this emphasis is not new – Malinowski himself made the same point – there is a real problem of how to give due weight both to individual autonomy and to the apparent existence of unified systems of symbolism and belief which seem to provide a framework for the activities of every member of the society.

One answer might be that these apparently overarching systems of symbolism and belief are in fact less pervasive than some accounts make them appear. There may be a wide range of beliefs amongst which members of a given society can pick and choose. Sholkamy describes just such a situation in an Egyptian village, in which the procreative beliefs of the local folk Islam – not entirely internally consistent themselves – face challenges from both modern medicine and the ideas of Islamic fundamentalists.

In this case it is not entirely clear how far a comparable range of intellectual choice has always existed, and how far the current situation is a product of rapid social change. This is an instance of a problem of interpretation that affects to some extent most attempts to understand traditional systems of procreative belief. The arguments which followed the Leach–Spiro debate about Trobriand procreative ideas (Leach 1966; Spiro 1968) brought in comments from many fieldworkers, and ranged from the implications of pig castration as evidence for understanding of insemination, to local theories of why a child might resemble its father without insemination (as locally understood) being involved. These debates encouraged other ethnographers to go on paying systematic attention to the issues raised by Malinowski. The kind of ethnographic data needed to settle the arguments can never have been particularly easy for outsiders to collect, and the difficulties increased since local beliefs have often been complicated or extinguished by the efforts of missionaries, particularly Christians, Muslims and the missionaries of progress in medical science. In modernizing states, the national educational systems, particularly the influence of medical teaching and family planning programmes, make major inroads into folk beliefs: it becomes ever more difficult to understand what people recently believed concerning these topics once their views have been defined as sinful, ignorant or both.

Nevertheless, there are powerful reasons for supposing that even the most traditional systems left considerable scope for individual interpretation. One reason for this is the very multiplicity of obviously traditional procreative metaphors existing within each society. This implies that while there may sometimes be a *prominent* metaphor, as that of the seed-and-soil in Delaney's Turkish village, we should not be quick to assume that it will prove to be a *dominant* metaphor, with the kind of ideologically hegemonic power to persuade that she argues for. For alongside one metaphor may be another, and alongside both there may be less metaphorical, more practical and proto-rationalist apprehensions, as when Thiessen's Macedonian women – resisting both the prevailing patrilineal ideology and the dogma that infertility must be accepted as God's will – secretly introduced a 'barren' woman to a man of proven fertility. And metaphors may exist, but apparently lack decisive resonance. The most explicit evidence for this view is the woman whom Thomas in chapter 2 quoted as answering his questions 'with patience':

> 'She continued: 'Women are "like flesh" (*akao nofitra*), they are "soft" (*malemy*); men on the other hand are "strong, like bones" (*matanzaka*, *akao taolana*), especially the backbone (*taolandamosy*), the strongest bone of all.' But this, she added, is 'only a way of speaking' (*fomba fiteny avao*).

Even more telling is Maia Green's demonstration in chapter 3 of how a single procreative idea can be socially manipulated in southern Tanzania. In the community she studied, female fertility is thought to depend on the provision of suitable medicines by men. But this situation, which might be expected to subordinate women to male control, is in fact flexible enough to allow almost any reproductive and residential choice a women decides to make.

Convincing as these examples are, they leave a feeling that the problem has been shifted rather than resolved. We appear to have moved from a rather caricatured image of traditional societies whose members unquestioningly accepted existing customs and the cosmological beliefs in which they were grounded – ignoring the obvious fact of individual autonomy – to perfectly valid analyses of automous action that leave us wondering how and why these cosmological systems arose in the first place. This is not a problem that can be resolved merely by saying that people are partly tradition-bound and partly autonomous. There is a genuine problem here which, despite the efforts of Bourdieu (1977) and others, we have no real idea how to resolve.

THE CURRENT STATE OF THE DEBATE

So where do matters stand today? Looking back at the earlier contributions, we can see that debates start over how far the role of the human male in reproduction was universally understood, and an exploration of the implications of a denial of the male role. The debate, under Leach's (1966) influence, then moved into the separation of official kinship and religious dogmas from more everyday factual knowledge, moving on to explore the implications of contradiction between two such ways of thinking. More recently, there have been attempts to grasp the cyclic linking of death and rebirth, and the conservation of human fertility under the social control of politically dominant groups and of religious authorities. From there it was but a short step to reveal the gender implications of metaphors which placed either men, or women in the most valued creative role at procreation. Where such foundational metaphors were strongly gendered, there proved to be connections to rights in land. Most recently the very role of symbolic systems has been called into question.

So far, then, the debates have retained some important threads, but have continued to shift ground. Nevertheless some progress has clearly been made, and the subject raises theoretical questions which are fundamental to the whole discipline of anthropology. We hope that the ethnographic essays collected in this volume will be seen both as interesting in themselves and as raw material for readers' own reflections on these fundamental issues.

These essays are also offered in the hope that the continuing analysis of procreation theories and their wider implications is a task with interest beyond the confines of mainstream anthropology. As Julia Stonehouse shows in chapter 11, social and symbolic concerns similar to those of so-called traditional societies have had a significant impact on the development of European embryological thought. Recent bio-medical and legal innovations in human fertility, such as in-vitro fertilization, anonymous sperm donors, surrogacy and pre-natal sex determination via amniocentesis, suggest that the potential for disjunctions between technical developments and existing social understandings is as great as ever.

The themes raised in this book are also relevant to the understanding of some purely social developments in modern society. British newspapers often carry harrowing accounts of child custody disputes known as 'tug of love' cases in which parents from two different societies each try to assert rights of control over their children. It is clear that in many of these we are witnessing not only the individual distress caused by a marriage which fails, but the additional anger and confusion which are likely to occur when a man from a society which believes that a single drop of semen carries an agnatic blood line, marries a woman from a society which has a more even-handed view of parental bio-genetic and social contributions. While such issues must be the subject of further research, the essays which follow will, we hope, help make them more visible and accessible in a world where more people than ever before might marry a partner from a different society.

However, changes in the social organization of fertility are not confined to such relatively marginal cases. In recent decades European fertility rates have tumbled, while in many countries the institution of marriage has undergone great changes, with rapidly rising divorce rates and dramatic increases in both cohabitation outside marriage and the proportion of children born within such relationships. The relationship between gender and economic activity has also been transformed. A hundred years ago, the interest of our intellectual forbears in exotic procreation arrangements was directly concerned with social and political developments affecting their own society. Does our own emphasis on the elements of flexibility in the procreative arrangements of exotic societies also reflect a need to understand how we can handle such developments in our own society? If so, this book is likely to be just one contribution to an ongoing debate with profound implications for us all.

NOTE

We are indebted to Maurice Bloch, Maia Green, Sini Cedercreutz, Maria Phylactou, Charles Stafford and Gill Shepherd for comments on this paper, but any errors or defects are of course our own. Peter Loizos would also like to thank Marios Sarris, Dimitris Theodossopoulos and Aigli Pittaka for collecting ethnographic material in Cyprus and Zakynthos which helped him forward with this volume. We would also like to acknowledge the stimulation provided by those who attended the original conference at the London School of Economics, in September 1996. They included Cecilia Busby, Janet Carsten, Terri Collins, Sarah Franklin, Joan Frigole Reixach, Bwire Kaare, Leonie Kindness, Heather Paxson, Sarah Randall, Nanneke Redclift, Todd Sanders, Dimitris Theodossopoulos, Gabriele von Bruck and James Woodburn. Thanks are due to the Suntory-Toyota International Center for the Study of Economics and Related Disciplines, at LSE, for funds which supported the conference.

CHAPTER 2

NO SUBSTANCE, NO KINSHIP?

PROCREATION, PERFORMATIVITY AND TEMANAMBONDRO PARENT–CHILD RELATIONS

PHILIP THOMAS

> To treat a specific characteristic of one particular culture as a feature of a fictive universal hardly seems wise to me.
> David Schneider

Since Rodney Needham (1971) and David Schneider (1972) effectively declared kinship to be a fiction of the analysts' making, there have been various attempts at rethinking the subject and calls for a reformulation of the problematic along with a new set of terms for analysis. This paper is in part concerned with two analytic terms which appear to offer much to kinship studies, namely 'substance' and 'performativity', and these are explored in the context of relations between parents and children among a people of southeast Madagascar. In short I argue that although Temanambondro recognize that 'fathers' and 'mothers' give birth to 'children', they do not think of this relation in terms of shared substance, nor do they view it as important or significant.[1] Instead, fathers and mothers are principally seen to be related to their children through ritually created relations and through the giving of 'nurture', both performatively constituted relationships. However, whilst the notion of performativity appears to offer a useful way of conceptualizing relations constituted through practice, I suggest that we need to pay attention in our analysis to the possibility that there are different kinds of performatively constituted relationship, and even different degrees of performativity. Following M. Strathern (1996), I also suggest that we need to be mindful of the possibility that what we understand as kinship may comprise a variety of ways of conceptualizing relatedness.

The ethnographic setting for the discussion of these issues is a people of rural southeast Madagascar who call themselves Temanambondro. Primarily subsistence farmers engaged in the production of wet-rice for household consumption, Temanambondro inhabit the lower reaches of the Iavibola, Isandra and Manambondro river valleys. Distributed among several villages ranging in size from 200 or so to one numbering 3,000 persons, Temanambondro comprise a ritual polity of a number of named 'ancestries' (probably in excess of sixty), each of which possesses a tomb located at the mouth of the Manambondro river. These groupings, often found in more than one village, are themselves divided into one or more discrete localized 'house-groups'. In the village in which I conducted fieldwork there were eleven named ancestries, the largest of which comprised twenty-eight house-groups, and the smallest only one. I leave aside a more detailed discussion of these groups until later in the paper. But for now I want to turn to look at what has proved perhaps the most influential approach in kinship studies over the past few years, the cultural approach of David Schneider, and examine in some detail one of its key analytic terms, the concept of substance.

RELATIONS OF SUBSTANCE

In recent years the field of kinship has seen a resurgence of interest, due in large part to contributions from the study of gender, personhood, sexuality and the new reproductive technologies (see e.g. Yanagisako & Collier 1987; Howell and Melhuus 1993; Peletz 1995; M. Strathern 1995; Weston 1995), and much of this work has explicitly drawn inspiration from Schneider's writings (e.g. 1968, 1972, 1984).[2] There are many strands to Schneider's work, but one of the most important concerns what he sees as the often unstated assumptions of what constitutes kinship.

In his critique of the 'conventional wisdom' of 'kinship' theory (Schneider 1984), Schneider argues that despite their differences almost all writers on kinship have assumed that kinship exists and then asked what does it *do* – a concern with its function – looking at its role in, for example, marriage, inheritance and the defining of social groups, or its use as an idiom for the representation of political and economic relationships. Rarely however has the question been asked 'what *is* kinship?' – a concern with its content – and, when it has, the tendency has been, either implicitly or explicitly, to view it as a socio-cultural elaboration on the 'natural facts' of biology and sexual reproduction; that is, *reducible* to birth and procreation.[3]

Rather than assume *a priori* what kinship is in any given instance, Schneider suggests that we instead ask such questions as 'what are the units, how are they defined in the native culture itself, how does it postulate their interconnections, their mode of differentiation, by what symbolic devices do they define the units of their relationship, and what meanings do these have?' (1972:58; see also 1984:181–201). It is therefore incumbent on the anthropologist to demonstrate rather than assume the value and significance of, for example, procreation, in a particular kinship system, and to show by careful ethnographic description how it is that a particular people conceptualize relations between people, something which they invariably do in a variety of ways.

Whilst Schneider's advocacy of a cultural approach to the study of kinship represents a fundamental reformulation of the problematic (see Schneider 1976), another of his major contributions is the introduction of the term substance into the analytic lexicon of kinship studies. The term is central to Schneider's 'cultural account' of American 'kinship', and appears in the context of a discussion of 'blood' relations, something which he contrasts with relations based on a 'code for conduct' (Schneider 1968:21–9). Since then the term has become something of a 'key symbol' in anthropological writings on kinship, and is frequently used as a shorthand for describing – in Schneider's terms – a mode of interconnection that native cultures themselves postulate.[4]

Although those seeking to 'rescue kinship from its post-Schneiderian demise' (Carsten 1995:224) are not always in total agreement with Schneider, many have found substance a highly useful analytic term and organizing metaphor. Indeed, Thomas Gibson has gone so far as to suggest that 'if we are to retain "kinship" at all as a cross-cultural category, we must restrict it to the comparison of the varying social implications of the symbol of shared physical substance' (1985:409). Whilst some may question whether a cross-cultural definition of kinship is possible, or even desirable, Gibson's proposal seems to me merely a strong version of a widely held assumption among those sympathetic to Schneider's views, namely that kinship is coextensive with the sharing, transmission and exchange of substance (e.g. Weiner 1982; Carsten 1995; Busby 1997a).[5] In short, cultural accounts of kinship frequently privilege substance such that it is seen as *the* key feature in the structuring of kinship relations.

Whilst I would accept that the term is not without its merits, and that some very sophisticated analyses of kinship in terms of substance have been made, I think there are also some problems with the use of the term. Aside from the fact that it risks perpetuating some of our own cultural preoccupations about the nature of kinship, as something rooted in bodies and conceptualized in terms of (ethno)biological processes, the term is sometimes used in such a way that it obscures rather than clarifies 'culturally posited forms of connectedness' (Schneider 1984:117). Occasionally references to substance do not contain sufficient ethnographic detail for the reader to clearly ascertain what the term signifies in a particular instance, and all too frequently the explanatory power of the term is assumed rather than demonstrated. Furthermore, even when the substance in question is specified it is not always clear how it is passed on or how it figures in the formation of persons and the conceptualization of relatedness.[6]

Another problem concerns the fact that substance is used to refer to a great range of things: not only blood (sometimes of different kinds), but also semen, as well as non-biogenetic material such as breast milk, food, medicines and even land. What unites these items is that they are directly or indirectly taken into the body – through conception, gestation and/or ingestion – producing the embodied grounds of shared identity. But given Schneider's insistence that we base our accounts on how people themselves conceptualize social relations and categorize different modes of connectedness, one wonders if, by referring to such disparate elements by the same term, there is not a danger of making local concepts superficially similar (although, *pace* Gibson, not necessarily comparable) whilst obscuring important differences in the way that these substances constitute relatedness.[7]

There is a rather delightful irony here given Schneider's theoretical and methodological position, as the word substance itself does not appear to have been one uttered by the 'natives', the informants of the Chicago kinship project. Schneider's claim that he *is* one of the natives notwithstanding, the term is in fact Schneider's own gloss on American ideas about 'blood' and 'shared biogenetic material' (1968:25). Admittedly the ethnography that arose from the project is little in evidence in *American Kinship*, for reasons which Schneider has elaborated on elsewhere (1980:123–4; Schneider and Handler 1995: 209–17), but still the fact remains that in many accounts of kinship, substance is not a native category but an analytic gloss offered to account for a number of different (and perhaps disparate) data.

That terms and concepts from one culture can prove useful heuristic devices in the study of another is unquestionable; anthropology is the proof of this (indeed, I hope this paper is too). But that they can be used unproblematically in this way is something of which we need to be mindful, for as well as opening up analytic possibilities they can also determine analytic perceptions. Too often discussions of substance pay too little heed to the particularities of specific substances. On this level then Gibson's (1985) proposal is dubious, for are 'substantial' relations necessarily comparable? On another level I think the proposal is misguided for it excludes alternative ways of constituting and representing relatedness, reducing kinship to a single principle and effectively leaving any society which does not imagine social relations in terms of substance without it.

To illustrate some of these points, let me turn briefly to a study from Madagascar: Richard Huntington's account of Bara personhood, gender and kinship (Huntington 1988). Basing much of his analysis on the implications of Bara procreation theory, Huntington discusses in some detail the substances contributed by mother and father during conception. Regarding the mother, Huntington tells us that 'the female transfers essential physical substance to the offspring' (ibid.:24), and adds that 'Bara view kinship ties through females as ties of biological substance relating to the event of birth' (ibid.:28). The substance in question appears to be blood, which Huntington says is ordered by the father's semen (ibid.:24). The significance of semen however appears somewhat ambiguous: the father 'contribute[s] some substance to the child, since it is specifically the semen that is responsible for conception' (ibid.:26), but Huntington goes on to say that,

> [a]lthough the accumulation of semen in the woman's womb is seen as one immediate factor in the conception and growth of the fetus, *this material link between father and child receives little emphasis in Bara idiom.* It is the formative action of the

> semen that is emphasized, *not* the transfer ... of material from father to child. (ibid., emphases added)

If this is so it is surely misleading to speak, as Huntington does, of a 'material link between father and child'. In fact his ethnography shows that relationships through the father are talked of by Bara in terms of 'ordering' rather than in terms of substance (ibid.:27–8). It is also unclear just how a mother's substance manifests itself in the child and how 'ties' of substance are understood by Bara, although at times, if somewhat equivocally, Huntington appears intent on arraying his data along the lines of the widely found model of female flesh versus male bones. This vagueness seems in no small part to stem from the lack of clarity of Bara views on the subject, and one wonders if Huntington is not guilty of over-intellectualizing what he was told, making much of a topic that Bara themselves do not see as central to kinship. Indeed Huntington's account is rather unusual given that many ethnographers have noted rather unsystematized ideas about procreation among other Malagasy peoples (e.g. Kottak 1980:311n.20; Astuti 1993:280–2; Bloch 1993:124–5).

As, however, Huntington is more explicit than some ethnographers about what he means by substance it is possible to analyse more thoroughly his use of the term. This proves to be rather interesting because it appears that there is an important difference in the way the two substances figure in the constitution of relatedness. For whilst a mother's 'blood' produces 'ties of biological substance', a father's semen apparently does not: the two substances thus do not form relationships of the same order. It is thus interesting to note that Bara are, in Huntington's terms, 'ideally [organized into] patrilineal and patrilocal ... corporate kin groups ... ordered on the uniquely agnatic relationship between the living and their immediate ancestors in the group's tomb' (1988:27, phrasing transposed). Shared substance then appears not to be the basis of Bara 'kin groups', and if the definition of kinship is to be restricted to relations of shared substance, what are referred to as Bara 'kin groups' appear not to be 'kin' groups at all.

Admittedly Huntington's discussion and use of the term substance is rather simplistic and confined to the analysis of local procreation theory. However, it does reveal particularly clearly how talk of substance may obscure rather than clarify local conceptualizations of relatedness, bringing to them a misplaced concreteness and purported naturalism that is a product of analysis rather than indigenous thinking. It also raises another problem, and one which I will focus on in the second half of the paper: what term(s) appear to be appropriate for analysing non-substantial relations, such as those which obtain between a Bara father and his children? Like Bara, Temanambondro do not imagine the relation between father and child in terms of substance. Instead, the dominant mode of representing the relationship is in terms of the ritually created relationship of ancestry and ongoing relations of 'nurture'. But before we turn to look at these relations I want to look in detail at Temanambondro ideas about birth and procreation, for it is here that I myself tried to discover whether Temanambondro imagined parents and children to be related through shared substance.

RELATIONS OF BIRTH AND PROCREATION

It is an anthropological truism that our research is shaped not only by the 'metacultural categories embedded in European culture' (Schneider 1984:184), but also by the debates and theories generated by our own and other disciplines. Inspired by cultural accounts of kinship, as I investigated the ways in which Temanambondro themselves conceptualized relations between people I sought to establish whether or not they did this in terms of ideas about substance. And to do this I began to look into the area to which virtually all accounts of substance make reference: birth and procreation.

As Gillian Feeley-Harnik has noted for an area of northwest Madagascar, birth 'is not inherently gendered' for 'both men and women "bear children"' (1991:67). Such too is the case among Temanambondro, and people speak of fathers and mothers as those who 'gave birth to' a child (*ñe aba niteraka anazy*; *ñe endry niteraka anazy*). There is some ambiguity about this, as we will see later, for fathers are also said *not* to give birth. But for the time being let us focus on relations explicitly connected to birth and procreation.

Although fathers and mothers give birth, the nature of the relationship is not at all clearly formulated as a relationship of inherited substance. A person is sometimes said to 'take after' (*manahaka*) a parent, in contexts of both character and appearance, whilst a more explicitly corporeal idiom is used to refer to the relation between siblings (and their offspring over succeeding generations), who are said to be of 'one stomach' (*troky raiky*) or less commonly 'one heart' (*tapo raiky*). On one occasion I heard the word *troky* ('stomach') used as a synonym for 'mother' when two people who had the same mother but different father were said to 'share the stomach but not share the father' (*miharo troky fa tsy miharo ray*). But when I asked what constituted relations of 'one stomach' and 'one heart', people tended to be rather vague. People of 'one stomach', I was once told, 'come from the stomach of their mother' (*avy tamin'ñe troky ñe endriny*), and on another occasion it was pointed out that both stomach and heart are 'inside' (*añaty*).

It would be easy to interpret these idioms as proof that mother-child relations are thought of as 'biological', but I admit to having reservations about doing so (cf. Astuti 1995a:97–8; see also Schneider 1984:79–92). Firstly, although a corporeal idiom is used to describe this relationship, the meaning of 'stomach' and 'heart' must not be taken for granted, and it is notable that people of 'one stomach' are not said to be of 'one womb' or 'one blood', those parts of the body mentioned in relation to procreation; indeed, I never heard anyone mention 'stomach' and 'heart' in this context. Furthermore, I think this idiom suggests more a concern with shared 'origins' than shared biology, a statement in keeping with culturally salient ideas about relationships between people in time and space.[8] At best I think we can therefore say that whilst there is perhaps some intuitive sense that people are connected through (in this context, women's) bodies, the exact nature of the relationship is left undefined,[9] a situation which also prevails with regard to procreation.

For Temanambondro, as for many Malagasy peoples, procreation remains a matter for conjecture, and when I asked about the topic I found nothing that could be called a local 'theory', only local speculation. In fact what people had to say about procreation tells us more about how people view the relationship that results in conception than it does about the physiological processes which lead to it. Those who had anything to say about the subject were usually women who were themselves mothers, but although men were less forthcoming on such matters nothing they said was in any way inconsistent with what women told me.

Everyone who was prepared to discuss the subject commented that a woman must 'lie' (*mandry*) with a man to become pregnant (*bevohoka*, lit. 'big womb'), and some pointed out that a woman has conceived when her period (for which there are various terms) 'does not arrive' (*tsy tonga*). Going beyond this a few suggested that the man's semen (again various terms) 'entered' (*misokatra*, *tafiditra*) the woman's womb and 'mixed' (*mifangaro*) with her 'blood' (*ra*). Beyond this however people said little, and when I asked how the child in the 'womb' (*trañon-daza*, lit. 'child's house') was formed the only person prepared to answer my question said that it was 'finished by God' (*vita Zanahary*).[10] In general, however, people's response to my questioning pointed to a lack of certainty on the subject, and several asked me if I knew what was involved (cf. Bloch 1993:124–5). But rather than view this as 'ignorance' of the 'facts' I see it as indifference. I think there is no clear theory about conception because it is not seen by people as terribly important.

Much more significant in my view is the way in which people spoke about the relationship between the woman and man who 'lie' together, using idioms strikingly similar to those employed to talk about what makes a successful marriage. This came through especially clearly in a conversation I had with two sisters, both in their 40s, who were happy to indulge me in talk about my bizarre interests.

Endrin'i Kako and Endrin'i Lavavolo both agreed that for a woman to become pregnant 'the man and woman must be the same' (*tsy maitsy mitovy ñe lelahy sy ñe apela*), they must 'follow one another' (*mifañaraka*). This idea of compatibility was also brought up to discuss 'blood'. Endrin'i Kako suggested that a man and woman's blood must be the same (*tsy maitsy mitovy ñe ra*); but Endrin'i Lavavolo countered with an example of a couple known to have different blood groups and yet who had children.[11] Perhaps blood groups do not have to be the same if the man has 'strength' (*heriny*), added Endrin'i Lavavolo, who then pointed out that if the woman has sex with a man only once the child may be weak and ill in its first months and years, and she cited an example in support of this. But Endrin'i Kako added that sometimes when a woman has conceived and then sleeps with a different man he may 'cause [the foetus] to leave' (*mampiala*). 'Isn't this because the first man and the second were not the same?' (*tsy mitovy*), she wondered aloud.

There are some interesting things to note about this conversation, which is typical of others that I had. Firstly, it seemed that for every nascent theory a countering example could always be found: local theory was thus being continually reformulated in practice. Secondly, the idea that blood groups do not have to be the 'same' if the man has 'strength' uses a metaphor which is frequently employed to define male things, something which we will see again presently. And finally, the idiom of similarity and complementarity, of things having to be the 'same' with regards to conception, is, as I mentioned, strikingly similar to how people talked about marriage. Similarity and complementarity are thus stressed as necessary in procreation and marriage. Indeed, the birth and growth of children is seen very much as completing part of the early stages of marriage, and a marriage that survives there being no children is very rare indeed.

In part pursuing a line of enquiry prompted by ethnographic reports of ideas about substance elsewhere in Madagascar and beyond, what I learned about conception did not appear very promising: a woman's blood and a man's semen seemed to be involved, but beyond that people had little to say, and did not seem particularly interested. Fearful however that I had perhaps missed something, I tried to find out more, this time asking questions about gestation and the body. Perhaps here I might find ideas about substance.

From noting what women did during pregnancy and asking questions about the child *in utero* I found out much, but not about substance. In fact it became obvious that, although people's concern for the unborn child focused on its susceptibility to a variety of environmental influences, these did not signal the presence of ideas about the transference of substance, but rather the transference of properties and qualities from an object to the child. As a result pregnant women were subject to a number of taboos, which all, however, point to concerns for the health of the child, rather than to ideas of transferred substance.[12]

Whilst quite explicit about such restrictions and the reasons for them, Temanambondro I discussed them with made no allusion to the effect of the mother's blood or a man's semen on the child during gestation that suggested any notion of a relation of substance between either parent and the unborn child. Finally, unable to think of anything but leading questions, I asked an especially eloquent friend whether there was an idea that 'blood' (*ra*) or 'flesh' (*nofitra*) came from the mother, and 'bones' (*taolana*) from the father, a claim made by one ethnographer and implied by another (Baré 1977:96; Huntington 1988:23–8). Explaining herself with patience, my friend replied, 'people sometimes say fathers "make [their children] strong" (*mampatanzaka*) and "give [them] strength" (*manome heriny*); whilst mothers give them "thought" (*hevitra*), "small talk" (*resaka madiniky*), and "nurture their self" (*miteza ñe fañahiny*).' She continued: 'Women are "like flesh" (*akao nofitra*), they are "soft" (*malemy*); men on the other hand are "strong, like bones" (*matanzaka, akao taolana*), especially the backbone (*taolandamosy*, alt. *hazondamosy*), the strongest bone of all.' But this, she added, is 'only a way of speaking' (*fomba fiteny avao*).

Of course an interpretation of these remarks revolves around what is meant by 'like' (*akao*): women are 'like' flesh, men are 'like' bones. However my friend did not say flesh 'comes from the mother' (*avy tamin'ñe endriny*), which would suggest something akin to the transference of substance, only that flesh is 'like' women; similarly she did not say bones 'come from' the father. Indeed, she said women 'give' children very insubstantial things: thought, small talk and nurture. Men meanwhile give them a quality, 'strength', not a substance. The gendering of 'flesh' and 'bone' is thus figurative rather than substantial, metaphoric rather than metonymic. Furthermore, it utilizes common metaphors for female and male qualities – 'softness' and 'strength' – applied in many different contexts (see Thomas 1996). Flesh and bones therefore exhibit gendered qualities, but they are not in themselves derived from inherited, transferred or gendered substances.[13]

To conclude the foregoing: whilst procreation and birth do create some type of relation, this is not thought of in terms of substance. Moreover, the relation is hardly elaborated upon and in fact does not constitute kinship in any significant sense; it 'counts for' very little (cf. Schneider 1980:120–4). The reason for this, I suggest, is that procreation and birth are not the template for Temanambondro kinship. Indeed Temanambondro place emphasis on relations constituted through practice rather than through procreation and bodily substances, as we will see presently. Thus we should not be surprised that they have no developed theory about procreation. A matter of no great significance, it is something good to do rather than good to think.[14]

DOING AND BEING: PERFORMATIVE KINSHIP

Despite their relative lack of interest in birth and procreation and the absence of a clearly articulated notion of shared substance, Temanambondro are very clear about the fact that parents and children are related. In fact a highly significant aspect of a person's social identity is derived from the relations they trace through their mother and father. Yet these relations are not premissed on notions of shared bodily *being*, but are instead constituted through ritual and other forms of social practice, acts of *doing*.

This distinction, between doing and being, derives from Schneider's analysis of Yapese relations between 'father', 'mother' and 'child' (Schneider 1984). Like Temanambondro, Yapese recognize a connection between coitus and conception, but as Schneider carefully demonstrates this fact 'is simply not culturally significant ... it [does not entail] the idea of ... shared substance ... [and] the Yapese definition of the relationship between *citamangen* ["father"] and *fak* ["child"] remains radically different from the European cultural conception of reproduction' (ibid.:73). What Schneider argues is that procreation, and the relationships between 'spouses' and between 'parents' and 'children', are conceptualized in terms of such things as 'work', 'exchange', 'care' and 'respect', actions which, instead of following already existing links of 'affinity', 'kinship' or shared substance, actually constitute the relationship.

Schneider's aim in contrasting doing and being is to stress how Yapese 'kinship' is not about relations of consanguinity or shared substance, a 'state of *being* [resting on] ... certain inherent and therefore inalienable attributes' (ibid.:72), but is rather about *doing*, 'role[s] ... performed' (ibid.:30). To some extent the opposition is a little overdrawn, and a number of examples could be cited which reveal substance to be acquired through ongoing social practice rather than merely from relations of procreation (e.g. A. Strathern 1973; Daniel 1984; Carsten 1995). However, the point I wish to emphasize here is that, with regard to Temanambondro, acts of doing *do not* produce relations of shared bodily being: social practice – be it commensality, shared residence or whatever – does not leave embodied traces or sedimented deposits of social relations in the form of shared substance.

In following Schneider's lead, rather than speaking of relationships as 'roles performed' I have chosen instead to speak of kinship as *performative* in an attempt to stress the ways in which it is (re)constituted through past and present practice. Although this sense of performative is not wholly consistent with that of speech act theory,[15] it is used in a similar sense to that of Sahlins (1985:xi–xiii, 26–31) in his discussion of 'performative structures'. Noting that 'customary kinds of acts can precipitate social forms as well as vice versa' (ibid.:xi), Sahlins suggests that performative structures are those which 'continuously mak[e] relationships out of practice' (ibid.:28). Kinship relations can thus be processually constituted through practice, rather than merely being the template for the organization of practice.[16]

A dominant feature of Temanambondro kinship is that it too is performative, constituted through ritual and other practices, such as exchange, as well as shared place, residence, work and consumption. The various relations constituted through practice are in turn represented in a wide range of categories and spatial, gendered, corporeal and botanical idioms and images. However, rather than try and present an exhaustive account of the varieties of performatively constituted relations in Temanambondro kinship, I want to focus here on two types of performatively constituted relation that exist between the categories of person that were the focus of the discussion of procreation, fathers, mothers and children. As we will see, these relations are not necessarily coextensive with those of birth, but they are far more significant and carry far more value nonetheless.

Relations of ancestry

As we have seen, a notable feature of what people had to say about procreation was the need for similarity and compatibility between a woman and man, one of the instances in which gender complementarity is emphasized. However, Temanambondro also make much of gender as a marker of difference, elaborated in a variety of ways and contexts, such as the division of domestic space, for example, and metaphors of 'softness' and 'strength' (Thomas 1995, 1996). Gender is also an important marker of difference in Temanambondro kinship, where relations traced through the father are thought of as quite different to those traced through the mother and other women (cf. Astuti 1993).

Although relations by birth are ideologically unelaborated among Temanambondro, connections between a person and their father and mother and other 'relatives' (*havana*) in terms of ancestry are much more clearly articulated. In Temanambondro terms, a person is said to have 'eight sides' (*valo ila*) or 'eight branches' (*valo sampana*), of which there are 'four sides with the father and four sides with the mother' (*efatra ila teña amin'ñe aba teña de efatra ila teña amin'ñe endry teña*). Each of these 'sides' is traceable to an actual person, and from the perspective of kinship theory the 'eight sides' represent a three-generation personal kindred (see figure 2.1).[17] However, Temanambondro tend not to talk about 'sides' in terms of individual 'ancestors' but rather in terms of the ancestry identity of the person they are related to and the place they 'came from' (*niboaka*). Thus talk of 'sides' is not of particular 'ancestors' but of relationships to collectivities and places traced through them.

Although Temanambondro do not number, order or rank the 'eight sides', 'the side of the father' (*ilan'ñe abany*) is referred to as the 'strongest' (*teña mahery*), and the father himself is known as the 'great trunk' (*fotora be*), the most important 'root' (*teña fototra*). It is through the father that a person receives their own ancestry identity, for 'the ancestry of one's father is one's own ancestry' (*ñe karazan'ñe aba teña de ñe karaza teña*), and the genderedness of this relationship is emphasized by the term used for those who are of the same ancestry: *lahiny*, from *-lahy*, meaning 'male'. By contrast, in relation to the ancestries traced through the remaining 'sides' – each constituted through relations with one or more women – the person stands as *anakapela*, 'child of women'. A person thus stands as *lahiny* to their own ancestry, and *anakapela* to all other ancestries to which they trace 'sides'.

In sociological terms, an ancestry is a named collectivity comprising a set of people of one or more 'house-groups' (*trañobe*, 'great house') who are said to 'have one tomb' (*mana kibory raiky*). Just as each and every house-group forms part (or all) of one and only one ancestry, so each and every person is *lahiny* of one ancestry. On the whole, those who belong to an ancestry are buried in its tomb, an event at which they are said to 'follow their father' (*miaraka amin'ñe abany*). But although the word *karazana* (which in the context of these named collectivities I have chosen to render as 'ancestry') derives from the root *razana*, meaning 'ancestor' (and also 'placenta'), the term itself is used more widely

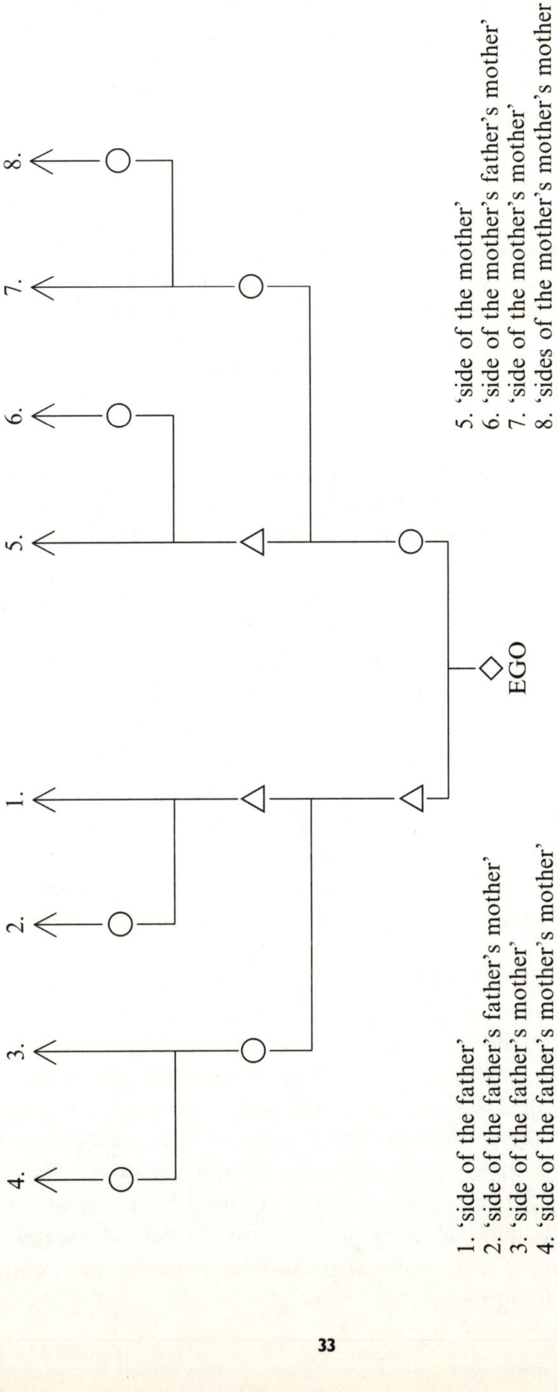

Figure 2.1 Genealogical representation of the 'eight sides' (*valo ila*)

to define 'kinds' of things, not only collectivities of people, but also species of trees, animals, cultivated plants, and so on. However, in sociological contexts the term *karazana* is not used exclusively to refer to groups who could be said to be related by 'common descent', and the term is better understood as a category which indicates a certain commonality among a class of things or people in contrast to another. Thus ancestries are, in Temanambondro terms, simply 'kinds of people' (*karaza'n̂'olo*).[18]

Received from one's father, one's own ancestry is however not an identity based upon birth, substance or a relation of 'descent' in the genealogical sense. Rather, it is an identity derived from ritual performance. This point was made clear to me by a man with whom I had many conversations, on this subject and others. Never one for plain speaking, Aban'i Betongatra began by telling me that: 'The mother carries [the child] for nine months and then holds onto the house post [when she gives birth]. The father, he simply collects firewood!' (*Minde sivy vola de mitaña andry ambo n̂e endriny. N̂e abany mila fotsivavo avao!*). He then sought to clarify this rather elliptical statement with a proverb: 'The shin bone does not give birth for custom makes (a man) have children in Manambondro' (*Tsy miteraka n̂e vaovitsy fa n̂e fomba mampananaka an-Manambondro*). The shin bone, he explained, is the 'father', and it is 'only custom that makes fathers fathers' (*n̂e fomba avao maha-aba n̂e abany*). The 'custom' in question is the *fafy*, the sacrifice of a zebu that marks the completion of marriage rites, and until this is done a man is not 'recognized' as being related to his children in terms of ancestry.[19]

Contradicting the idea that a father is simply someone who 'gave birth to' a child, this formulation of the father-child relation explicitly points to the idea that it is not coitus that makes a man a father but a ritual. On completion of this rite a man becomes the father of all children subsequently born to his wife, and his children thus take on his own ancestry. In the context of this relationship, a father is said 'to give a name' to his children (*manome anarana*), the name of his own ancestry, and to gain 'recognition' or 'law' (*adidy*) with respect to them. The reason for the rite is to explain to the ancestors that such-and-such a man is the father of his children;[20] effectively it performatively creates a man as a recognized father of the children born of his wife, just as it performatively creates his children's own ancestry identity.

A conventional interpretation of this situation would be to argue that the marriage rite is concerned with the legitimation of relations derived from procreation, such that the 'social' relations between a father and his children are based on a template of 'biological' relatedness. What I want to argue, however, is that this is not the case, and that relations of ancestry are not an elaboration on the 'natural facts' of reproduction but a different kind of relatedness altogether. To establish this we need to look in more detail at some of the ways in which men can make themselves fathers of children.

Take the following three scenarios. Among Temanambondro it is not unusual for a man to marry a woman who already has a child. Upon completing the marriage rites, the man may negotiate with his 'in-laws' (*rafoza*) to have the child 'recognized' as his own regardless of whether or not he is known to be the father who 'gave birth to' the child. Indeed it is sometimes well known that he is not, but if the child is subsequently 'recognized' as his own then he becomes the child's father and the child takes on his ancestry identity.

A practice known as 'buying the iron with the handle' (*mivango vy amin'ñe androñany*) also clearly demonstrates the irrelevance of procreation to relations of ancestry. For Temanambondro, to be childless is considered an affliction deserving of compassion, and people often give up their own children to be fostered by close relatives. But for a man, the situation is seen as especially grave, for without children (and especially without a son) he is said to be 'dead and done for in [his] house-group' (*maty tanteraka ampatrange*). Men too may foster, but up until recently a man with few or no children would sometimes choose to marry a woman who was pregnant, although by whom was unimportant. Before she gave birth the marriage rites would be completed, and so the man became 'recognized' as the father of the subsequently born child. Having struggled to produce them, in 'buying the iron' (the woman) 'with the handle' (the unborn child) the man could be more certain of having children who would survive him.

Whilst this practice establishes a father's 'law' before the birth of his children, the completion of marriage rites also extends that 'law' beyond its lifetime. Whilst there is some ambivalence about making such claims nowadays, it was formerly the case that a man would be 'recognized' as the father of any children born to his wife within three years of his death, or within the same period if the couple had separated but not divorced. A child born during this time is known as a 'child of law' (*zanak'adidy*), because until a marriage is formally terminated it is said that 'there is still law' (*mbola misy adidy*).[21] Again the man becomes the father of the child despite the fact that he is known not to be related to it by birth.

Each of these three scenarios clearly illustrate how relatedness by birth is irrelevant to relatedness by ancestry: fathers may be related to their children by birth, but in theory it does not matter if they are not, for completing marriage rites, or 'finishing custom' (*vita ñe fomba*), is what 'makes' men into fathers. This can also be seen in the context of children born of unmarried women, who are said to 'have no father' (*tsy mana aba*).[22] Children who 'have no father' are hardly a new phenomenon among Temanambondro, although their numbers appear to be on the increase due to economic factors concerning marriage rites (which need not trouble us here). These children are also known as *zanak'adrao*, 'children of the *adrao*', born of men who typically pass by a woman's house at night but are gone in the morning, just as the *adrao* (a nocturnal 'wild cat') prowls at night but is never seen in the day.

Whilst said to 'have no father', *zanak'adrao* could also be said to have two different fathers. Firstly, they have a father who 'gave birth to' them. Importantly, however, this father has not 'given' the child a 'name', for the child is not of his ancestry. In fact the child takes on the ancestry of their mother, or more accurately their mother's father, who stands to them as another kind of father. For although *zanak'adrao* are of their mother's ancestry, a relationship which appears to derive from birth, in terms of the 'eight sides' the child is incorporated into their mother's generation, such that 'the side of the father' is that of the mother's father, and 'the side of the mother' that of the mother's mother.

The rather ambiguous position of *zanak'adrao*, who have two fathers and yet 'have no father', stems from the fact that they have no father who has 'finished custom' with their mother. This ambiguity extends to what is a virtual denial of the significance of birth in the constitution of ancestry, for their own ancestry is represented not as that of their mother but as that of their mother's father who stands to them as father in terms of the 'eight sides'. One could say that so long as no man 'finishes custom' with his 'daughter', the 'law' he establishes at his own marriage extends over her children too. Thus the ancestry of the *zanak'adrao* is represented not as due to birth, but due to their mother's father having 'finished custom'.

This suggestion is in keeping with the dominant mode of representing relations within ancestries in male terms (cf. Bloch 1987). Indeed, as it is men who perform the rite that completes marriage, it could be said that men are the ones who (re)produce ancestry, and the contribution of women to this process is systematically marginalized through denial of the importance of relations by birth and procreation. Yet just as fathers are not simply made by birth, neither are mothers, and although mothers are not made by 'custom' they, like fathers, can make themselves through another type of performatively constituted relation, the giving of 'nurture'.

Relations of 'nurture'

Relations of ancestry are particularly important in contexts of ritual, inheritance and the defining of marriageability and incest; they are in effect the 'structuring structures' (Bourdieu 1977) of social reproduction and inter-generational continuity. Fathers, mothers and children are, however, also performatively related through the giving and receiving of 'nurture' (*fitezana*). Like ancestry, relations of 'nurture' do not always coincide with relations by birth; but unlike ancestry, 'nurture' is a largely ungendered relation, constituted in contexts of everyday practical existence, in the intimate, familial and familiar world of the household, and in ongoing relations of work and consumption, of farming and feeding.

One way of understanding the importance placed on relations of 'nurture' is to look at the practice of teknonymy.[23] Having children effects an important status transformation among Temanambondro, making people into 'adults' (*olombe*), a state denoted by a change of name whereby the person becomes known as 'father of X' or 'mother of X' (*aban'i X*, *endrin'i X*). Teknonyms are a form of 'respect' (*haza*, *hasy*) and 'honour' (*voniñahitra*), and although there is some variation in the practice, it is common for them to refer to the first-born or eldest surviving child, regardless of gender. Teknonyms also signal an ongoing and reciprocally constituted relation of 'caring for', 'bringing up' and 'nurturing', all glosses on the verb *miteza*. In the context of teknonymy fathers and mothers thus performatively make themselves through giving 'nurture' to their children and 'making them grow' (*mahabe anazy*). This is also the case for those who are childless and who make themselves fathers and mothers by fostering, a relationship similarly defined as one of 'nurture', for foster parents themselves acquire a teknonym, becoming known as father or mother of the child they foster.[24]

I once heard it said of a woman fostered by her mother's childless brother that she had 'made living' her mother's brother's 'name' (*nahavelo ñe anarany*), for, it was explained to me, 'if [one] doesn't have children then one's name dies ... and [becomes] lost' (*laha tsy manan'anaka de maty ñe anarany ... de laha maty de very*). A teknonym then is a 'living name', born of another living person, signalling a living relationship of life-sustaining 'nurture'. But there is also the issue of memory here, about the way in which, despite being dead, one's name is not 'lost', tantamount to being forgotten. Frequently ancestors who 'did not give birth' (*tsy niteraka*) are rendered nameless, by not being 'called' during ancestral invocations, for example.[25] A person's 'name' is thus remembered through association with those in succeeding generations who were 'made living' by that person's 'nurture', and their continuing to flourish and live 'makes living' the 'name' of those who 'nurtured' them, ensuring that it does not become 'lost'. Thus, even though a man is said to be 'dead and done for in his house-group' if he does not have children through whom to be remembered, he may still foster or 'nurture' children, and their presence in the world will ensure that his name does not 'die' and become 'lost', but is instead remembered and thus 'made living'.

The giving of 'nurture' is thus another way in which parents and children are related performatively, and, in the case of fostering, a way in which men and women can make themselves fathers and mothers outside relations of birth and ancestry.

CONCLUDING REMARKS

The cultural approach of Schneider has proved highly influential in the recently rejuvenated field of kinship studies, and my own analysis of Temanambondro notions of relatedness is heavily indebted to it. However, unlike many working within this tradition, I have not found the concept of substance a useful one, for reasons which I hope are now clear. To take Schneider's own contrast, I have tried to show how – with regard to relations between fathers, mothers and children – Temanambondro emphasize the importance of 'doing' over ideas of bodily 'being', making kinship primarily performative rather than substantial.

But, whilst the notion of performativity appears to offer a useful way of conceptualizing kinship relations which prioritize performance, practice and process over procreation and corporeality, 'as [it] begins its ascent ... as an analytic paradigm' (Morris 1995:586), is there not a danger that the term harbours the same problems I highlighted regarding substance? There appear to me to be at least two issues here: one concerning the conceptualization of kinship; and the other, the conceptualization of performativity.

Anthropological studies of kinship have frequently attempted to isolate a core principle upon which all relations of kinship are premissed or based, an obvious example being Gibson's (1985) suggestion that kinship lies in the symbol of shared physical substance. This attempt at purifying kinship has recently been criticized by M. Strathern, who (following Latour 1993) has suggested that kinship is in fact always a hybrid, a heterogeneous set of principles for reckoning relatedness, in which '[o]ne kind of reckoning never operates alone; it *always operates in conjunction with* factors of a different order. From the anthropologist's comparative viewpoint, "kinship" has to lie in the combination' (M. Strathern 1996:530). Although the implications of her remarks cannot be gone into in detail, Strathern's point is highly relevant to the context which I have been discussing, for Temanambondro imagine at least three ways in which fathers and mothers are related to their children: through birth, ancestry and 'nurture'. Furthermore, by disaggregating these three modes we can see that none is the template for the others; each is *different from* rather than being *derivative of* another. There is thus no essential principle to Temanambondro kinship, and although I have suggested that Temanambondro kinship is primarily performative, non-performative relations by birth are also recognized, although deemed to be of little significance. In our analyses of the conjunction and combination of different modes of reckoning relatedness we therefore need to examine carefully the ways in which these modes are interrelated and the contexts within which one mode is prioritized over others.[26]

Regarding the second issue, it is a notable feature of Temanambondro kinship that there are different types of performatively constituted relationship, and different degrees of performativity (cf. Ahern 1979). To appropriate Temanambondro gender metaphors for my own ends, the rite that completes marriage could be said to be a 'strong' kind of performativity: once a man has performed it, his children's ancestry identity is determined once and for all and cannot be changed. The rites accompanying birth and death – burial of the placenta in the house-group compound; disposal of the umbilical cord in the river; and burial in the ancestry tomb – are not actions which performatively reconstitute a person's relation with their own ancestry but merely reiterations of the already established relation.[27] On the other hand, relations traced through the mother and other women could be said to be 'weak' and subject to eventual forgetting. This is less so with the 'sides' of the mother and father's mother than those of more distantly related women – such as the mother's mother's mother, father's father's mother and so forth – to whose own ancestry a person stands as *anakapela*. These relations need to be continually reconstituted, something which primarily occurs through participation in rituals which function in part as a 'technology of remembrance' (Morris 1995:576). During these rituals cattle are killed and butchered, their meat divided among the participants, and nowhere is the fact that these rituals involve performative acts of remembering more clearly demonstrated than in the name for the small bundles of meat given to *anakapela*, known as 'histories' (*tantara*). Finally, relations of 'nurture' are similarly weak, reconstituted through everyday acts of caring, and enduring for those who foster not in the categorization of ancestry but in their teknonym.[28]

The notion of performativity is attractive because it appears to offer a way of talking about the manner in which certain relations are made or repeatedly remade through practice. Furthermore, at least in Madagascar, it seems to capture something of a more general cultural principle for the constitution of persons, relations and identities.[29] But we need to constantly keep in mind the potential of our analytic terms and methodological strategies to obscure as well as illuminate. As I have suggested there may be degrees of performativity and varieties of doing that we need to distinguish. Furthermore, performativity does not characterize the whole of kinship: it is not that being and doing are necessarily mutually exclusive principles, nor in the present case that one produces the other. Rather, taking being to denote relations by birth rather than substance, both are present and co-exist, one a dominant and the other a subordinate principle within the hybrid which comprises Temanambondro 'kinship'.

NOTES

The research on which this chapter is based has been funded by the Economic and Social Research Council (UK) and the British Academy. Fieldwork in the Manambondro region of south-east Madagascar was carried out between December 1991 and October 1993 and undertaken under the auspices of the Musée d'Art et d'Archéologie/Institut de Civilisations of the Université de Madagascar, Antananarivo, in collaboration with the Ministère de l'Enseignement Supérieur and the Ministère des Affaires Etrangères of the Democratic Republic of Madagascar. I am grateful to all these institutions for enabling me to carry out my work. This is a revised version of the paper originally presented at the workshop at LSE and later given at the Social Anthropology seminar at UCL in October 1997; participants' comments on both occasions proved highly useful. I am additionally grateful to Jennifer Cole, Gillian Feeley-Harnik and Karen Middleton for commenting on different aspects of the paper, as well as to Peter Loizos for his encouragement and forbearance. Cecilia Busby commented on successive versions of the paper and made countless suggestions as to how they might be improved; her analytic insight and encouragement has proved once again invaluable. My thanks also go to my Temanambondro hosts, and in particular to those among them who found time to talk to me about procreation and relatedness, including Aban'i Rezy, Aban'i Bina, Endrin'i Vohira, Endrin'i Marie and Endrin'i Rikako. Needless to say I alone remain responsible for any errors of fact and waywardness of interpretation.

1 For ease of reading I have not used inverted commas for the terms 'father' (*aba*), 'mother' (*endry*) and 'child' (*anaka*, *zanaka*) but ask the reader to keep in mind the fact that these terms are meant as glosses of local terms and do not necessarily imply a status derived from relatedness by birth. As will become clear, for a person to be a 'father' or 'mother' does not necessarily entail their 'children' being related to them by birth.

2 Although Schneider's work has proved highly influential it has not met with unequivocal support (e.g. Scheffler 1991; cf. Schneider 1984:113–132), and even those broadly in sympathy with his arguments have not hesitated to point out some of their shortcomings (e.g. Yanagisako 1978; Carsten 1995). Schneider is perhaps most open to criticism regarding his theorization of culture, an issue that cer-

tainly merits discussion but which cannot be gone into here.

3 For a useful discussion of the significance of procreation in the anthropological study of kinship and gender, see Franklin (1997:17–72).

4 Use of the term substance has proved highly influential in discussions of kinship in Melanesia (e.g. Wagner 1967; A. Strathern 1973; Clay 1977; Weiner 1982; LiPuma 1988) and India (e.g. Barnett 1976; Inden and Nicholas 1977; Daniel 1984; Busby 1997a; cf. McGilvray 1982); use of the term, however, is by no means confined to these regions: see also e.g. Gibson (1985) and Carsten (1995).

5 Although some have used it outside the context in which it was originally formulated, Schneider himself has questioned the universal applicability of the contrast between 'substance' and 'code for conduct', pointing out that the opposition is specifically one of American culture (1980:120). With regard to 'substance' itself, although he makes no comment on the use of the term by other ethnographers, in his reanalysis of material from Yap Schneider is especially clear on the fact that, whatever Yapese 'kinship' might be, it is not a relation of shared 'substance' (1984:72–3 *et passim*).

6 Illustrative of these points is Gibson's (1985) own account of Buid relations of shared substance, where it is not at all clear what substances are contributed by either parent to the formation of the child, either at the time of or subsequent to conception (1985:399); nor is the uncertain nature of substantial relations helped by an unexplained contrast between 'physical and spiritual substance' (ibid.:391). For similarly vague examples from Madagascar, see Bloch's discussion of the Merina term *havana* (1981:7) and Kottak's account of Betsileo sibling terms (1980:202); both authors speak respectively of shared and gendered substances without elaborating on the nature, meaning, value or significance of these.

7 For an illuminating discussion which highlights the contrasting ways in which substances make relations in India and Melanesia, see Busby (1997b).

8 This concern with 'origins' is also articulated in terms of 'roots', and the word for 'heart' (*fo*) is one of a number of cognate terms involving these ideas. On Temanambondro concern with 'origins' and 'roots', see Thomas (1996, 1997).

9 Interestingly, as do all Malagasy, Temanambondro prohibit marriage and sexual relations between children of two sisters. Those who offered explanations for this 'taboo' (*fady*) tended to emphasize bodily connectedness: children of two sisters are of 'one stomach', they have often shared the same breast. In fact, apart from children of two sisters, anyone else related as people of 'one stomach' are not only permitted to marry, they are also preferred marriage partners (see Thomas 1996: ch. 6). Similarly, those who have shared the same breast may also marry as long as they are not children of two sisters. When pushed on these points people gave up and simply said children of two sisters were 'too close' (*akaiky loatra*). Again, I would suggest that reference to bodily connections to explain the marriage

prohibition between children of two sisters points to an intuitive sense of some form of corporeal relatedness, but the nature of this is not clearly formulated.

10 The phrase 'finished by God' comes close to what we mean by 'natural', although I only ever heard it used to describe the physical form of things, such as the foetus in this case and a rock formation in another.

11 Knowledge of the existence of blood groups has entered people's conceptual universe through State and Church medical services. It should be noted however that the significance of 'blood' to the two sisters is not necessarily the same as it is to you or me: there is nothing inherent to blood that determines its meaning, and here the significance of blood concerns the compatibility of similar kinds rather than ideas about shared substance.

12 There are a large number of such taboos, of which the following are highly illustrative. For example, a man should not bring his pregnant wife firewood entwined in vines, lest the child emerges at birth entangled in its umbilical cord; similarly, a pregnant woman should not sit on an upturned mortar in case the child is born with a 'broken' head. A number of foods are also tabooed, such as those classified as 'cold' (women are kept 'hot' during and after pregnancy), and many women abstain from others (such as avocado, jackfruit and honey) which are understood to block the child's orifices. For a comparable discussion of environmental influences and taboos regarding birth, see Bloch (1993).

13 Apart from investigating ideas surrounding procreation, I also looked into whether food and land could be seen to produce relations of substance. This proved to be an even less fruitful line of enquiry than investigating procreation.

14 The absence of ideas about shared substance and a relative lack of interest in procreation are broadly in line with a lack of elaborated concern with the body in Temanambondro notions of the person, at least when seen from a comparative ethnographic perspective. Personhood is instead formulated more around concepts of 'mind' (*saina*) and the 'moral self' (*fañahy*), the latter an aspect of being which only emerges in humans to make them 'living people' (*olombelona*) a month or so after birth. Before then new-borns are known among other things as 'animals' (*biby*). On Temanambondro concepts of person more generally, see Thomas (1996).

15 The term performative originates in Austin's (1962) theory of speech acts. In anthropology the notion of performativity has proved especially useful in the analysis of ritual (e.g. Tambiah 1981), and more recently in gender studies (see Morris 1995).

16 It is noteworthy that I have found the work of both Schneider and Sahlins helpful in analysing Temanambondro data, for, like myself, both are writing about Austronesian peoples. However, lest it be mistakenly understood that we are dealing with a phenomenon peculiar to this cultural cum linguistic grouping, see Witherspoon's discussion of Navajo kinship, in which he states that '[a]lthough the Navajo

believe that through sexual intercourse and birth some kind of common substance is shared ... [they] never mention common substance in finding or invoking kinship ties or norms. Kinship is discussed in terms of the *acts* of giving birth and sharing sustenance' (Witherspoon 1975:21, emphasis added).

17 'Sides' traced to a woman may also be represented in terms of the relationship with the woman's brother, e.g. the 'side' of the father's mother is also known as that of the father's mother's brother; this is in keeping with the general principle of viewing relations of ancestry in male terms (see below).

18 For discussion of these 'kinds' elsewhere in Madagascar, see e.g. Bloch (1971:42–3), Feeley-Harnik (1991:23–6) and Astuti (1995a).

19 Space precludes a description of the rite here. For a discussion of this and other Temanambondro marriage practices and rituals, see Thomas (1996: ch. 6).

20 My paraphrasing of a friend's explanation: *izany ne dikany ne fafy: manazava amin-drazana ty lehilahy ty de ne abany ty zaza ty.*

21 It is possible that the notion of *adidy* in relation to marriage emerged during the colonial period in the context of enquiries into the juridical dimensions of marriage and/or as an outcome of the fact that many men experienced long absences from their ancestral homeland during periods of labour migration. Unfortunately I am unable to verify whether or not this is the case.

22 For comparable discussions of the plight of persons born outside marriage in west Madagascar, see Astuti (1993) and Feeley-Harnik (n.d.).

23 For a comparable discussion of teknonymy in the context of parent-child relations, see Bloch (1993).

24 There is no verb 'to foster' or a separate term for 'foster parent'; Temanambondro merely speak of a person who fosters a child as someone who 'nurtures them' (*miteza anazy)*, something they distinguish from a person who has 'given birth' (*niteraka*) to their child. Although fostering is not lexically marked as a distinct form of 'nurture', I have chosen to use the term 'foster' for ease of exposition.

25 Similarly, when I collected 'genealogical' information I frequently found that, although the gender of ancestors who 'did not give birth' was usually remembered, their names were sometimes forgotten. It was by checking names gathered in 'genealogies' against names 'called' during ancestral invocations that I discovered that childless ancestors were frequently not 'called'. As these invocations are one of the primary means by which ancestors' names and identities are remembered, neglecting to 'call' certain ancestors is one way in which they, and their names and identities, will eventually be 'lost' and forgotten.

26 I hope to more fully explore the implications of Strathern's paper elsewhere in an analysis of the ways in which different modes of reckoning figure in the context of disputes over the ways that fathers and mothers are seen to be accountable for the actions of their children. This will emphasize how such relations are constituted and

negotiated in practice, whilst the current emphasis is on their structural logic.

27 Temanambondro thus differ from other Malagasy peoples where this identity is said to be determined by burial (e.g. Bloch 1971:45; Huntington 1988:35–6; Astuti 1995a:88–9); even when a person is not buried in their own ancestry tomb, this does not change their ancestry identity.

28 Of course the performative constitution of relations can co-exist with their deconstitution, through annulment and denial. Although this is certainly an important feature of Temanambondro 'kinship' it is one that I cannot go into here.

29 For other discussions of performativity in Madagascar, see Lambek (1992) on taboo and personhood, and Astuti (1995b) on non-'ethnic' collective identity. Interestingly, both authors view kinship, and what they choose to call 'descent', as non-performative (Lambek 1992:259; Astuti 1995a:3 *et passim*), a position at variance with my own.

CHAPTER 3

PROCREATION THEORIES AND THEIR IMPLICATIONS

OVERCOMING THE ABSENT FATHER IN SOUTHERN TANZANIA[1]

MAIA GREEN

INTRODUCTION

This article gives an account of some aspects of ideologies of procreation and the ritual practices with which they are associated among communities defining themselves as Pogoro in southern Tanzania. Human fertility and reproduction are viewed as part of a life-long process, which is not complete until the children born to a couple are themselves adult and capable of reproducing. The successful completion of this process ultimately depends on a woman's relationship with two men in successive generations: her father and the father of her child. Human fertility as an inherent capacity of the person is insufficient in itself to ensure successful reproduction. A person's latent potentiality for fertility has to be socially augmented. This is achieved through the ingestion and application of substances classified as 'medicines' (Green 1996), as well as through special practices which safeguard and augment the reproductive potential of women.

Although maternity as a relationship between a mother and her children is conceptualized as a 'natural' consequence of gestation, birth and suckling, paternity as a social relationship must be created through the incorporation of medicines, as well as payments for rights in the children of a particular man. This relationship is pivotal because of the representation of paternity as the catalyst in human reproduction. The reproductive potential of an individual woman depends on the incorporation of special medicines provided by her father. The ideological emphasis on paternity, however, is not manifested in social practice. As in other parts of Africa, many women are not married, and female-headed households constitute a significant proportion of any particular community (Clark 1984; Sender and Smith 1990; Omari 1995). Children born of short-lived unions are said to have "no fathers". In such cases, even where the father is known, he will not be identified by the mother, and the child adopts the names and family identity of his mother's fathers and brothers.

Local theories of procreation, kinship and descent, like the metaphors through which they are articulated, do not determine social practice in any immediate way (cf. Strathern 1973:25). Anthropological accounts which prioritize the kinds of kinship ideologies expressed in ritual and formal contexts may give a misleading impression of an unproblematic continuity between ideologies and practice. The apparent continuities between ideologies and practice are often artefacts of specific historical processes which effect the categorization of bounded domains of practice as 'tradition' or 'custom' (cf. Falk Moore 1986; Kratz 1994:321). These processes are clearly evident in the domain of kinship, where anthropologists have long been at pains to point out the considerable gaps between formal ideologies of kinship and how people actually negotiate relationships on the ground (cf. Bourdieu 1977; Schneider 1984). Among Pogoro communities in Ulanga, paternity as both status and social relationship is not simply ascribed to the genitor of a child. The social role of father may be assumed in practice by the mother's father or brother. A range of social practices can be accommodated by the local theory of paternity because it is constructed, like all kinship relations, as pre-eminently social. This flexibility raises important questions for rethinking the relationship between kinship practices and kinship ideologies in relation to gender. It also points to the significance of female autonomy for the practical constitution of kinship and descent (cf. Parkin and Nyamwaya 1987:4–5).

ECONOMY AND SETTLEMENT

The people defining themselves as Pogoro are a group of Bantu-speaking[2] agriculturalists with an estimated population of some sixty thousand, who occupy the central part of Ulanga District, southern Tanzania. The communities resident in the villages where I conducted my fieldwork in the early 1990s occupy a highland area of forested river valleys and grow maize, hill rice, bananas, sweet potatoes, groundnuts, cassava and beans. With the exception of a few wealthy individuals, they did not keep cattle or goats. The bulk of the highland population had been moved into nucleated villages under the Tanzanian government's villagization programme in the 1970s. This resulted in a shortage of good agricultural land in areas immediately surrounding villages (Maghimbi 1990:258). By the late 1980s many families had returned to pre-settlement homesteads. Seasonally split residence between farm and village was common. Within designated villages residential land is allocated by village governments, who also have the power to allocate agricultural land within village boundaries. In practice, customary tenure applies, and long-established plots are inherited from relatives or lent out to kin and neighbours. Although land in rural parts of the district was generally not bought and sold, renting arrangements, often of one season's duration, were widely entered into, especially in parts of the district where productive land was scarce.

Groups of related households tend to build close together. These groups usually centre on a group of brothers, joined by widowed, divorced or unmarried sisters, their adult children and spouses. In the ideal, the people who share a dwelling are a man, his wife and young children. In reality, household composition is fluid and constantly shifting around a residential core (cf. Guyer and Peters 1987). A person's relatives have latent rights to food and hospitality. The closer the relationship the greater the rights to reside. Siblings, parents and children, real and classificatory, may turn up and stay for months, if not years. Ultimately, such shifts of residence are constantly renegotiated as new households form and fragment. Some shifts are partial. Young men may sleep in one house and take their meals in another. The fostering of children is not unusual and long-term visiting is practised when food is short.

MARRIAGE

Conjugal relationships are worked out in progressive stages, which may, or may not, include an official state-recognized marriage, usually in a Catholic church (Green 1993). As long as bridewealth payments have commenced, and a man and woman are living together, they are locally accepted as husband and wife. Marriage is conceptualized as virilocal, emphasized by the expression *kamtola* (he took her), which connotes the constitution of practical marriage. In practice, choice of residence is negotiable. A man may settle with his wife's kin if there are economic advantages in so doing, at least in the short term.[3]

Marriage transactions in much of Ulanga have undergone dramatic transformation throughout the twentieth century. Whereas brideservice, combined with the transfer of wealth objects to the bride's kin, was the norm until the 1940s, this system has been progressively replaced by the conversion into cash of the labour and wealth items previously exchanged. The payments now transferred to the bride's family are referred to generically as *maheto* (hoes), in reference to the wealth items which supplemented brideservice in the past, although the Kiswahili words **posa** and **mahari** are often used.[4] *Maheto* consists of a series of payments which continue to bear reference to either the objects or the labour which were previously exchanged. This determines, in part, its division. A portion of cash called *matemeko*[5], representing the brideservice component, goes to the person or people who stand in the relation of parents to the bride. Specific payments are made to persons standing in the categories of bride's mother's brothers (**mjomba**), her mothers, and father's sisters (**shangazi**).[6]

Maheto payments are made in successive instalments over an extended timeframe (cf. Parkin 1980). They are not finalized until several years after the woman has gone to live with the husband, and children born. Although a married woman is usually buried at her husband's place, she never loses her connection with her natal family, to which she may well return in the event of his death or a separation.[7] And, while the component payments made to specific categories of the bride's kin recognize her mother's role in her upbringing, compensate her parents for the loss of her labour and for her removal, and give her husband legal rights to her offspring, these are by no means absolute. The consent of the woman's brothers is needed prior to her marriage, and a child may choose where to make his or her home, settling more or less permanently at the place of either their mother's or their father's relatives (cf. Gluckman 1950:171).

Marriage, however, is not the determining feature of Pogoro kinship. I estimate that approximately one-third of households are female-headed, due to a combination of divorce, widowhood, choice and male labour migration. A high proportion of marriages end in separation. Practical divorce is fairly straightforward, entailing the reversal of practical marriage, the woman returning to her place and to her natal kin. Bridewealth payments may be returned if separation occurs early and the woman has not borne children. The separation of the parents does not alter the relationship between parents and children. Nor does it terminate ritual obligations between spouses. Even those who have formally divorced are obliged to shave at the funeral of a former partner. As in other rural African communities, adult mortality rates are high. With an average life expectancy at birth of around 45 years, the death of a spouse is common. Widows are less likely to remarry than widowers, although they may well have informal partners and boyfriends.

The relative ease of separation and the option for women to establish their own matrifocal households seem to have been characteristics of Pogoro kinship for much of the twentieth century. District records from the British colonial period remark on the high proportion of female-headed households, even in the 1930s, and the fact that many marriages terminated prior to the completion of bridewealth. Where women became pregnant prior to betrothal or marriage, children remained with the mother and were the legal responsibility of her fathers and brothers.[8] Similar arrangements were certainly practised by other groups occupying the regions between south western Tanzania and the coast, at least from the late nineteenth century to the 1960s (Beidelman 1967). This flexibility was interpreted by early observers as being due to the inevitable collapse of what were perceived to be matrilineal kinship systems, characterized by marital instability and the dynamic of competition between husbands and wives' brothers (Richards 1950; Beidelman 1967:xiv; Swantz 1970:88; Poewe 1978). In reality, the majority of these peoples seem to have recognized both matrilineal and patrilineal descent as alternative succession options, and different attributes and kinds of property were passed along relatively shallow patrilineal and matrilineal lines. The ease of separation and the option for women to live with brothers and sustain their own households seem to have been an intrinsic feature of this kind of system, rather than an index of radical social transformation.

Of course, there have been changes. What appears different about the contemporary situation is not so much the incidence of female-headed households or marital instability, as the perception of some women that bringing up children alone is a positive choice in a context where the advantages of marriage, particularly for women, are ambiguous. All too often marriage for women simply means having an additional adult to support, whereas for men it is the only way in which they can establish a household of their own. The majority of resident men over the age of about thirty-five have wives. Men are reluctant to marry early. As any child can be claimed whether a man is married to the mother or not, a man can have the status of fatherhood without the burden of a wife, and can usually obtain for free from a sister the kind of domestic services that a wife would be expected to provide. While men aspire to having long-term live-in partners who may become wives, marriage is less essential for women. This is mainly because an adult woman can create and sustain her own household without recourse to a husband. She can perform agricultural tasks alone or hire in male labour where appropriate. As the domestic division of labour centres on women's contribution, men need access to female labour for cooking and food preparation if they are to avoid the humiliation of performing what are locally viewed as female tasks.

Whereas an adult man without a wife or children cannot really have a functioning household, a woman can achieve this through her children. Having children gives a woman status as an autonomous adult and enables her to create a household around them. Adult people are known by teknonyms, indicating status as a parent, rather than spouse. Marriage is desired by young women as a goal to aspire to, but being married is not the defining feature of female morality. What is shameful for women is to be 'rotten' (**bovu**) and barren. Illegitimate babies are greeted with enthusiasm by single mothers, especially if the child is a boy. Many such children are named **Bahati Njiani** – 'Luck on the Path'. Women who do not marry or have a permanent relationship with one man, for whatever reason, tend to form their own matrifocal households and choose to keep some of their children for themselves. Whereas in the past these children would have been the formal responsibility of a woman's brothers and fathers, mothers now have *de facto* parental responsibility for their own children, except on formal ritual occasions. If a woman consents, other children may be given over to their fathers if a payment is made.

ASYMMETRICAL EQUIVALENCE AND THE QUESTION OF DESCENT

Attitudes towards property or the social construction of property relations have implications for the extent to which ideologies of descent are realized in social practice (Worsley 1956; Bloch 1975). For peoples like the Pogoro, without cattle and with a flexible system of land tenure premised on usufruct rights, descent has little practical relevance for social organization. A person has multiple identities and potential affiliations to those to whom they are related (*walongu*) scattered over a wide area. The core of significant kin encompasses those related through the mother and through the father, their own offspring, grandchildren, siblings and the offspring of siblings. Crises such as funerals or events such as marriage bring kin together as transient groups, the constitution of which depends very much on the occasion. Kinship is dramatized at funerals and relationship marked out by such actions as shaving, marking the faces of the relatives of the deceased with flour, the transaction of various token payments and the inheritance of property and names. Participation counts, as 'evidence of kinship' (Wilson 1957:200) but, because there are no absolute rules determining the categories of kin who participate, and because of the expansive and classificatory nature of kinship (cf. Radcliffe-Brown 1950:8), Pogoro kinship is essentially pragmatic and open to manipulation, with no emphasis on descent groups as such.

Like other southern Tanzanians, Pogoro people differentiate between practical kinship and the ideologies of descent which are articulated and enacted in formal contexts such as the giving and receiving of bridewealth, matters of inheritance, and rituals surrounding processes of reproduction and death (cf. Wilson 1950). On these occasions descent is made explicit as the basis of certain rights and obligations between people standing for each side of a family, and the acknowledgement of certain symmetries between them. A person traces descent from both their mother's people (*washimau*) and their fathers' people (*washitati*). In the event of offerings (*tambiko*) to 'remember' the dead, identical sets of offerings are set out for each side, that of the mother and that of the father. Deceased members of both patrilineages are invoked to come and partake of the food, drink and, occasionally, pieces of cloth set out for them. On the father's side, this includes the father, his brothers (who are also classificatory fathers) and their fathers, and on the mother's side, the mother, her brothers and fathers. Pogoro people, like the Kaguru, construct their relationships with the dead around the eldest living descendant, who makes offerings to the parental generation on behalf of junior siblings (Beidelman 1986:11).

Recognition of both the father's people and the mother's people in the context of *tambiko* offerings is not an indication of double descent. On the contrary, the inclusion of the mother's brothers is a logical consequence of adelphic succession in which younger brothers succeed elder brothers and an elder son inherits the position of his father, dividing same-generation siblings across generations by transforming elder brothers into 'fathers', conceptualized as an office or status. While this construction of descent privileges the mother's patrilineal kin, it permits recognition of what appears as a limited matrilineal option across adjacent generations from mother's brother to sister's son (ZS), facilitating the transfer of paternity, as a social relationship, to the matrilineal line. This is possible because a brother and his sister are equally related, whether descent is reckoned patrilineally or matrilineally. The inheritance of names and statuses can, and did, pass either from father to son or from maternal uncle to nephew.

There is much debate today among people in their fifties and sixties about the proper principles of descent and succession and the relative importance of the maternal uncle's rights as opposed to those of the father.[9] According to older people, until the early years of this century the mother's brother had extensive rights over his sister's offspring, at least some of whom could expect a share of his inheritance. The maternal uncle had the right to sell one of his sister's children into slavery in times of famine, without the consent of the child's father, although the father's rights over his other children were uncontestable. The possibility of alternative reckonings of descent in matters of inheritance and marriage transactions certainly confused the colonial authorities who attempted to make patrilineal descent legally binding in January 1935.[10]

The debate over the relative positions of fathers and maternal uncles now has limited practical significance. Succession to positions of shrine mediumship continues to pass from maternal uncle to nephew (*mpwa*), but, where a paternal relationship is recognized, the inheritance of immovable property such as new brick houses passes from fathers to sons. Formal kinship transactions and the etiquette of avoidance and respect stress the potential equivalence and practical asymmetry of maternal uncles and fathers. In some ways the father and the mother's brother are equivalents, as the male representatives of the two sides to which an individual is related. Yet equivalence here does not imply equality, but asymmetry. The two positions are not conceptualized as equal, but as alternatives. One position or the other must be emphasized. This asymmetry is dramatized in the etiquette of respect and in funeral and marriage payments. On formal kinship occasions the father and the mother's brother are represented as alternative sources of male authority associated with rights over the allocation of property and persons.

Marriage and funeral payments are divided among specific categories of kin on both sides of a person's family, that of the father and that of the mother. If a woman was living with her father's kin, the bulk of the payment is handed over to those standing in the social position of father, while the male representatives of the mother's family receive only token payments. If a woman lived with her mother's kin the pattern is reversed, and the bulk of the payment goes to a mother's brother or, if he is alive, her father. The ambiguity of descent is perpetuated by the fact that many women do not marry and continue to live with, or near to, their brothers. If they have children who are not claimed by their fathers, these children are, and were, affiliated to the group of their mother's father.[11] The mother's brothers of these children then assume the office of 'father' on formal occasions, giving the impression that it is indeed the mother's brother who, in certain contexts, has a considerable degree of influence over the offspring of his sister.

The complexity of Pogoro reckonings of descent defies the convenient anthropological categorizations of *either* patrilineal *or* matrilineal descent systems as unbroken chains of continuity, traced unilineally through ascending generations. Rather, Pogoro people emphasize the possibility of alternate reckonings of descent between adjacent generations of living people, parents and children. This explains why, when Pogoro reckon descent for matters concerning the dead, the emphasis shifts again to the patrilineage of the mother through her father (who is also her brother's father), and not her mother's brother.

CLOSENESS AND RELATEDNESS

The asymmetrical equivalence of mother's brothers and fathers is further justified by notions of relatedness, conceptualized in terms of degrees and kinds of closeness premised on the sharing and embodiment of different kinds of substance. Although a person's mother's sisters and father's brothers are also classified as 'mothers' and 'fathers', birth parents are differentiated from their siblings. Similarly, siblings related only through one parent are differentiated from those born of the same parents (cf. Wilson 1950:114). Siblings born of the same father and mother are thought to be especially close, and the 'one father, one mother' nature of their relationship is emphasized. Those related only through the same father are thought of as being somewhat less close, although this is played down in formal contexts such as the handing over or receiving of bridewealth, or on other occasions when brothers want to present a united front to outsiders. Because a woman may have children with several different men over her reproductive lifetime, and because men move between relationships and a minority are polygynous, it is not at all unusual for siblings to be related through only one parent.

Offspring of the same father have a different kind of closeness than offspring of the same mother, who are said to have been 'born from the same belly' or 'suckled at the same breast'. This gives the latter a kind of 'natural' closeness, an idea of maternally related kin which extends to encompass all those related on the mother's side who are classified as *walokolu*, as opposed to merely *walongu*, a term for generic kin which also refers to those related on the father's side. The special closeness of maternal kin stems from the fact that maternity as a social relationship is regarded as uncontestable and given, as the biological template on which other kinship relations can be constructed (cf. Astuti 1992). In contrast, paternity is conceptualized as a social relationship which has to be created through the transmission of substance via the medium of kinship medicines, as well as payments for rights in the child.

BLOOD TIES

Notions about biological paternity and maternity are vague in some contexts and more elaborate in others. In conversations on this subject, adult men and women maintained that it is the man's 'blood' (*mwazi*) or 'seed' which forms the foetus. The woman is merely a belly, whose role is analagous to the soil in which a seed is planted. Younger people gave greater weight to a woman's role in reproduction, talking in the graphic imagery derived from primary school textbooks, likening the woman to a hen with eggs inside its body or a gun loaded with bullets. Among all age groups opinions differed regarding the extent to which the woman's blood enters into the substance of a foetus. Some men eventually conceded that it must all get mixed together when the child is in the womb, but others doggedly maintained that the foetus is formed solely from the 'blood' of the man.

This insistence makes sense when we consider the significance of notions of 'blood' in Pogoro constructions of kinship. 'Blood' is an idiomatic reference to semen, to the biological contribution a man makes to a child, but it also refers to family, to those to whom one is related.[12] The former understanding of blood informs the cultural epidemiology of a disease known as *mapinga,* to which women who conceive after sex with more than one man in fairly close succession may fall victim. *Mapinga* is caused by the mixing up inside the woman's body of the 'blood' of all the men with whom she has been sleeping. The symptoms of this disease are said to resemble epilepsy (**kifafa**), which is highly visible in the area (Jilek-Aal 1979:616). The foetus is also affected. Such pregnancies, it is said, never come to term, or if they do, the mother never survives the delivery. Under the British administration, the symptoms of *mapinga* were taken as evidence in native courts that a woman was committing adultery, for which her husband could claim compensation[13]. Although younger women now dismiss the risk of *mapinga,* it continues to haunt the imagination of elders who are keen to encourage female kin whom they suspect of sleeping around to seek medicine to prevent the onset of the disease.

The ideas underlying *mapinga* strongly suggest that 'blood' should not be mixed up and should go only one way, from men to women. Thus not only is it considered unclean for a man to sleep with a woman during her period, it is also considered dangerous, as the blood entering his body may make his genitals swell. These ideas are consistent with the statement that the blood which makes the foetus comes from the father, and the woman is nothing but a vessel. However, the implications of these notions are not pushed to the limits of the kind of logic behind them in the justification of categories of marriageable kin. People say that not only did they marry cross-cousins in the past, but that this was a preferred union. A man could marry either his father's sister's daughters or his mother's brother's daughter (real or classificatory). Despite the fact that notions about blood would seem to imply that the offspring of the mother's sister are of the same degree of unrelatedness as either cross-cousin, the marriage of parallel cousins, as classificatory brothers and sisters, was prohibited.

Notions about blood and biological kinship run on two apparently contradictory levels. On the one hand are notions about 'biological' blood and the mixing of it. On the other, 'blood' is an idiom for the conceptualization of relationships, which can be created through exchange but must be augmented with medicine. These two aspects of 'blood', as common substance and as a symbol of social relations, are present in the idea of blood brotherhood, which was, according to the older generation, previously practised. When people say 'this child is his blood', pointing to a child's father, they also say 'this child is his wealth'. The two expressions are used interchangeably. They can also refer to a pregnancy. The woman 'has' (is with) the foetus (*kana inda)*, but the *inda* itself belongs to the man who has responsibility towards it. Mothers of pregnant teenage daughters try to make their daughters tell them who the father is, 'because then if we know, we can go to him and say (pointing to the girl's belly), "This is your *inda*. Look after it"'. Pogoro notions about 'blood' as constituting kinship suggest that, even if we take into account notions of folk biology (cf. Carsten 1992:45), kinship is not solely about blood in any inherent 'biological' sense.

Children are a person's 'wealth'. This is especially emphasized for men, with whom rights in children traditionally lie. Social relations and obligations continue to be regarded as wealth. Although people in their twenties and thirties are beginning to see children as a cost, as rural living standards plummet and the price of education rises, the pauper remains the person without kin, rather than the person without property. In a practical sense children are wealth because they are labour and because they increase a person's network of kin, but children are a man's 'blood' and a man's 'wealth' because the man has given wealth over for the child. This is either as bridewealth *(maheto*) for the child's mother, or as a one-off payment to her relatives for rights in the child. It is this payment which makes the child formally the child of that father and his fathers. Yet this payment itself, like conception and birth, is insufficient to create paternity as a social relationship between a man and his children without the giving of medicine after the child is born.[14]

CREATING PATERNITY

Like other peoples the world over, Pogoro people make explicit comparisons between the fertility of plants, animals and people. A newborn's umbilical cord is planted like a banana sucker in a clump of banana trees by an old woman who is past childbearing age. This is done in secret, to prevent others from displacing the cord and stealing the fertility of the mother. The cords of baby girls are planted at *ndala*, 'female' banana trees, which produce many small fruits and reproduce quickly. Those of boys are buried at banana trees considered 'male', yielding big, heavy fruits with fewer bananas to a head.[15] Plantlike natural fecundity in itself is an insufficient basis for the reproduction of people. A man as a person has 'no root of the family', so he has to create it with medicine made from roots[16].

Babies are given a medicine called *shirala* before they can be taken out of the house inside which they have been secluded with their mothers until the tied end of the umbilical cord drops away. This medicine ensures that a man's children will 'grow' and become fertile adults. It also ensures the fertility of his daughters. This medicine should be provided by the child's father and is made from the ground roots of a tree, which, in the ideal, come from his ultimate place of origin and have been handed down for generations. If a family has no *shirala* medicine, it can be bought from a specialist who knows where in the forest to collect it. This medicine is applied to specific places on the child's body. A small quantity is put into the child's mouth. Although each family has slightly different ways of applying the medicine, what is important is that the medicine is rubbed on the child's body and consumed by the child. The medicine is thus incorporated by the child, just as the child itself, through the consumption of the medicine, is incorporated into its father's side. If a child has 'no father', that is nobody claiming the social position of father, the medicine comes from the side of the mother's father.

The medicine for babies is ground by both the child's parents from two pieces of root. One of these is big and fat, and is called *mdala*, 'woman'. The other, small and thin, is *mpalu*, 'man'. The symbolism here relates to sexual intercourse, with which grinding and pounding are associated (cf. Beidelman 1964:370). Each parent grinds his or her own root into a powder which is mixed with water to make a paste which will adhere to the child's body. A man should not see his first child of each sex of a particular union until he, together with the child's mother, has put the medicine on the child's body. He should do this with his eyes closed. 'Seeing' is a way of talking about knowledge, particularly knowledge of the relationships between things, events and people. Only after the child has been given *shirala* by the father can the father see his first child of each sex of that particular union, and only after the child has been given the medicine can the child 'come outside' of the house. The connection between paternity, as the child's relationship with the father's side, and the coming out of the house is explicit. *Shirala* here transforms the baby into a socially recognizable being, as the child of somebody, who can come out of the house and into the wider society. Like the 'ikipiki' medicine of the Nyakyusa, it not only marks the relationship between the child and the father's side, but *creates* it. As one of Monica Wilson's informants explained, 'They say of the medicine it is our kinship, it is our blood ... The medicine is to create relationship' (1957:105).

Although maternity as an immediate social relationship between mother and child is imagined as being somehow natural, female reproductive capacity ultimately depends on medicine from the father. While boys receive *shirala* medicine only once in their lifetime, girls are given another dose when they reach puberty, as, without it, they will be unable to have children. Should one of their offspring die while they are still living, they are again given the medicine, or their fertility will be impaired for ever. *Shirala* medicine is given to girls on the occasion of their first period, during the events leading up to the *unyago*, the instruction, seclusion and coming out of girls. The complex series of ceremonies and rituals which comprise the *unyago* have two main objectives. The first is to 'teach' (**kufunda**) the girls and transform them into potential wives and adults, as others have remarked on for the similar rites performed for girls throughout east and central Africa (e.g. Richards 1939, 1982; Beidelman

1964, Swantz 1966, 1970; Turner 1968; Caplan 1976; Brain 1978). Secondly, and more importantly, the rites aim to make the girls fertile in a direct and immediate way. Without their proper completion girls will either be infertile, as among the Zaramo (Swantz 1970:365) and Nyakyusa (Wilson 1957:101), or, as among the Bemba (Richards 1982:124) and Ndembu (Turner 1968:200), they will have difficulty in reproducing.

Female fertility is achieved through the giving of another dose of *shirala* medicine, in addition to a specific fertility medicine made from ground cucumber seeds (*ntanga*). The *shirala* facilitates reproductive capacity. The *ntanga* are used to absorb excess fertility and stop it seeping away (Green 1993). Consequently, the *ntanga* are initially eaten only by the girl herself and older women past sexual activity who can absorb this capacity in their bodies and prevent others from stealing it. After about a week, when the girl's state has been stabilized through various procedures which centre on washing and cooling her body, the *ntanga* are publicly eaten without restriction at the girl's coming out ceremony.

Pogoro people conceptualize reproduction as a long-term process which encompasses the growth and maturation of offspring. Proper reproduction maintains the proper order of adjacent generations, in which parents die before their offspring. The death of a child while the parents are still living is represented as an affront to the fertility of the parents. Special funeral practices are performed for the first child of particular parents to die while those parents are still living (*mjindu*). Mourning is forbidden. The funeral lasts only one day. After the burial the child's mother is given another dose of kinship medicine to restore her fertility in a ritual which transforms the funeral into a collapsed re-enactment of the girls' puberty rites. At the end of the day the parents of the dead child are supposed to resume sexual relations.

OVERCOMING THE ABSENT FATHER

Pogoro ritual practices centring on fertility and kinship emphasize the social construction of paternity, while formal kinship occasions stress the role and position of the father. Despite the seemingly 'natural' connection with maternal kin, the asymmetrical opposition between father and mother's brother generally privileges the father on occasions when formal kinship is enacted, except in cases where a person has 'no father' and is thus only matrilineally related. The paternal relationship is fundamental to the realization of social reproduction. Human reproduction is conceptualized as involving a complex sequence of social and biological relationships in which the successful development of a child in the woman's womb and outside it depends on her relationship with two men in different generations: her father and her sexual partner, who may or may not become her husband or the social father of her child. The provision of *shirala* for a child by a man creates paternity as a social relationship between father and child, assigning the child to its father's family and to their place of origin. It ensures that children grow and that girls will be fertile, sustaining the fiction that without the tangible contribution of substance from the father's side the child would be weak, and that the fertility of women depends, in part, on socially recognized relationships through men.

In contrast to the reality in which many children 'have no fathers', paternity is represented in ritual contexts as *the* pivotal relationship on which social reproduction depends. The absence of a patrilineal father, however, does not necessarily imply the absence of a paternal relationship. Pogoro paternity is based on two principles: the incorporation of kinship medicines and land substance, rather than semen, and on rights over persons rather than impregnation. It follows, therefore, that the mother's brother can assume the social position of the father through the acceptance of social responsibility for his sister's offspring and the provision of *shirala* medicine from her father's place of origin. Paternity conceptualized in this way can, and does, skip generations, and the role of father and the substance he provides can be assumed by a woman's father or brothers. Marriage is not the only means of establishing a paternal relationship with a woman's children. Indeed, while marriage is aspired to by most people as a kind of universal ideal, the realities of death, separation and short-term unions mean that marriage is frequently a temporary state for both men and women.

The manipulability of paternity rests in part on its conceptualization as a pre-eminently social relationship. Similar constructions are found among other peoples throughout much of Africa, where the distinction between pater and genitor is pronounced, and where a woman's illegitimate children are incorporated into the lineage of her father or, alternatively, if she has a husband, into his lineage group (Parkin 1980). Pogoro people are less preoccupied with legitimacy than some of these other peoples who are more concerned with descent groups as corporate property-holding bodies. This is partly due to their particular constructions of property relations in which groups use land and resources, rather than hold them, and in which livestock do not constitute a corporate resource for the reproduction of kinship relations.

Another factor, underplayed in many accounts of African kinship, is also significant (cf. Molyneaux 1977; Harris 1981). This concerns a perception of women as autonomous adults who have strong complementary relationships with men as brothers and with other men as husbands. Although a woman's fathers and brothers receive substantial portions of bridewealth payments, and although formal marriage is represented mainly as an exchange between the men from the bride's and groom's family groups, a woman who leaves her husband is welcomed home by her brothers and fathers, and cannot be forced to remarry. It is not unusual for homestead cooperating groups to consist mainly of separated or bereaved brothers and sisters and their children. Loyalties between husbands and brothers have to be constantly negotiated (cf. Beidelman 1986:12–18). As among the Digo of coastal Kenya (Parkin 1980:215), women play a significant role in these negotiations, largely because they do not need husbands or brothers to establish their own households and become the core adults in matrifocal family units.

The discourse privileging paternity and the relationship with men on which human fertility depends is enacted in practices which give it a temporary reality of a most fleeting nature. While women acknowledge the importance of *shirala* medicine for human fertility and growth, they point out that their children do not need a father for this, as their own father can provide the medicine in his place. When women talk of human fertility they place greater emphasis on the special protective practices which are the responsibility of women: the preparation of the *ntanga*, the *unyago* and the maintenance of the various prohibitions on pubescent girls and post-partum mothers. A social relationship with a husband or the father of one's child is not then essential for social reproduction. Nor is it necessary for the establishment of an autonomous household or family group. The crucial factor is the relationship with a woman's 'father' who has provided her with medicine. Of course both men and women acknowledge the importance of biological factors in the process of human reproduction, irrespective of the transmission of medicines, but what is important is the fact that the biological act is insufficient in itself to produce offspring without first ensuring the fertility of the woman with a combination of medicines and various puberty and post-partum practices.

KINSHIP THEORY AND KINSHIP PRACTICE

Pogoro constructions of relatedness and reproduction can be viewed as either radically divergent from social practice, or as an ideological system which flexibly accommodates a range of practices without having to dramatically reconstitute itself. The former interpretation is consistent with the theoretical orientation of the kind of Africanist anthropology which invented African kinship as a unique system, premised on descent groups and marriage as the transfer of women between them. This view of African kinship prioritized the given nature and immutability of descent. Despite the evident ambiguities of paternity as a social relationship in many African systems, birth was, nevertheless, seen to determine fundamental identities between offspring and parents (Fortes 1953:30; Bloch 1992). Structuralist accounts focused on formal relations between descent groups, expressed through marriage transfers and the genealogical reckonings on which ancestor cults depended. Studies of ritual as a special formal domain of meaning-generating activity supported the accounts of formal kinship, obscuring the ambiguities of everyday social practice as a different kind of reality, one lacking the authenticity of what ethnographic analysis constituted as the formal system.

Yet, despite relegation to the inauthentic, everyday social practice emerges as a clear contradiction to formal systems, even in the older African ethnographies. Among the Nuer, for example, descent groups had minimal significance for the organization of daily life in villages and cattle camps (Evans-Pritchard 1940), while the matrilineal peoples described by Richards pursued such a range of descent, relatedness and marriage strategies that the 'puzzle' Richards perceived (1950) emerges largely as an imposition of the ethnographer (cf. Schneider 1984:vii). That the gap between what people did and their formal accounts of it was enormous did not escape the attention of either anthropologists or colonial administrators. The most obvious explanation seemed to lie in the radical changes brought about by the incorporation of rural communities into the colonial order and global economy. African kinship was viewed as fragile. What were thought to be 'traditional' systems were described as being on the verge of collapse, an interpretation supported by the discourse of the male elders, the main beneficiaries of kinship institutions, with respect to control over women, juniors and property resources. Colonial administrations responded by codifying customary law and constructing a formal domain of 'tradition' (Ranger 1983).

There are, however, more plausible explanations for the lack of correspondence between social practice, anthropological theories and local ideologies, both historically and in the present. The most obvious is that neither anthropological theories nor local ideologies are representations of reality in any simple sense. While such theories are 'models of' and 'for', in Geertz's sense (1973:93), they remain a model, and, moreover, a model constructed by both parties from a restricted set of components. This set for Africa conventionally includes descent groups, jural rights and obligations, ancestors and ritual. While models can be built with relative ease using these components, living people on the ground work their way around the set pieces, changing, amending, manipulating, tracing descent in any number of ways, repositioning ancestors and shifting genealogies. Compromise and flexibility are the core features of social life in any society, past and present. The notion of 'tradition' subscribed to by anthropologists and informants alike on certain occasions obscures this fact deliberately, conveying a false impression of a past which is not only without history or change, but which is threatened by it. This is not hard to comprehend if we accept that notions of 'tradition' are themselves political and constitute part of a legitimating framework in the societies which routinely invoke them (cf. Ranger 1983; Boyer 1990). Consequently, when people talk about 'tradition' they are making statements about the present, rather than describing the past, and are generally doing so in terms of rigid models of the way things were, and by implication ought to be. These 'traditional' constructions are often identical to the kinds of ideal models anthropologists create. Both tend to serve particular interests, privileging males, for example, or high-caste viewpoints, or particular constructions of ethnicities in a similar ideological way (cf. Moore 1995:35). Disjunctions between local ideologies and what people actually do cannot be explained simply in terms of historical transformations on a static past. Social practice is never wholly determined by models and metaphors, although it may be justified by them retrospectively (Kratz 1994:321). Although Pogoro ideologies of social procreation stress the male contribution, local practice is flexible, precisely because relationships are not given but socially created. Ritual and formal ideologies do not determine social practice, but on the contrary, can accommodate a range of possibilities.

NOTES

1 This paper is based on twenty-one months of fieldwork in Ulanga District conducted between 1989 and 1991. The original research was funded by the UK's Economic and Social Research Council. The Tanzania Commission for Science and Technology kindly granted research permission and the Department of Sociology at the University of Dar es Salaam provided additional support. Two short visits in 1995 and 1996 were made possible by the University of Manchester. I am grateful to the people of Ulanga District for their hospitality, assistance and cooperation.

2 Pogoro people, like other Tanzanians, speak a local language, Kipogoro, and the national language, Kiswahili. Both are Bantu languages. Kipogoro terms in the text are italicized, Kiswahili terms appear in bold. Terms which are the same in both languages are italicized in bold (as in ***mjomba***).

3 Probably until the 1960s this strategy was associated with poorer men, who were more likely to have performed longer-term brideservice rather than convert the brideservice component of bridewealth into cash.

4 Hoes seem to have been a common wealth item for marriage exchanges throughout central, southern and coastal tanzania until the 1930s, according to the accounts in Beidelman (1967).

5 From *-temeka,* to do brideservice, to clear grasses.

6 The **mjomba** receives a payment called *shilemba*, after the turban or piece of cloth which he could previously claim. Some families today give a blanket rather than cash. The *shangazi* is entitled to chickens, or cash in lieu, while the mother of the bride receives a payment called *shibebeo*, after the carrying cloth in which the bride was carried as a child.

7 Caplan describes a similar situation for the Swahili of Mafia Island and its implications for female autonomy (1976).

8 The District Book hints at the instability of marriage as early as 1934, when many marriages collapsed before the completion of the bride-

wealth and the children remained affiliated to the family of their mother (Morogoro (Eastern Province) Provincial Book vol. ii: Bagomoyo and Ulanga District Books, Microfilm MF17,TNA).

9 Swantz (1970:88) and Beidelman (1967:xiv) describe similar debates among Zaramo, Kaguru, Luguru and other peoples occupying south western and eastern Tanzania.

10 The General Rule set on 1 January 1935 states that the primary heir who is responsible for the distribution of a man's property and wives 'shall be a man's brother NOT his son or *mpwa*, and if no brother it shall be his son and not *mpwa*' (see Mahenge District Record Book, in Morogoro (Eastern Province) Provincial Book vol. ii: Bagomoyo and Ulanga District Books, Microfilm MF 17,TNA.

11 This trend appears to have been long established by the 1930s (see Mahenge District Record Book, in Morogoro (Eastern Province) Provincial Book vol. Ii: Bagomoyo and Ulanga District Books, Microfilm MF17,TNA).

12 As MacCormack points out, many of the terms used to talk about kinship and procreation are polysemous, conveying a range of associated concepts and ideas, from the physical to the cosmological (1982:126).

13 See Mahenge District Record Book.

14 See Aijmer (1992:10) for an account of Nyakyusa post-birth kinship practices. He states that, 'The Nyakyusa forge links between the new individual and the universe of kinship not in terms of sexual intercourse or conception, but only after the birth of the infant' through 'ikipiki medicine'.

15 The banana symbolism of the Nyakyusa is very similar, with plantains equated with the male and sweet bananas with the female (Wilson 1957:37–8,106).

16 Among the Vezo of Madagascar paternity is also conceptualized as a relationship which must be socially created, in contrast to 'natural' maternity (Astuti 1992).

CHAPTER 4

MAKING PERSONS, MARKING DIFFERENCE

PROCREATION BELIEFS IN HIGHLAND BOLIVIA

ANDREW CANESSA

INTRODUCTION

Procreation beliefs are frequently highly illuminating in understanding how relations between persons are conceived. Descent is often articulated in terms of shared substance and so it seems clear that examining procreation beliefs will shed some light on how people understand kinship ties. But descent is not always considered in lineage terms and not always rooted in something as concrete as blood or bone. Descent can also be conceived in terms of a shared relationship with generalized spirits or even place: descent can be a shared belief in one's autochthony. In such cultures, too, procreation beliefs shed light on how people relate to each other but relatedness may be processual and dynamic rather than rooted in immutable substance. Moreover, relatedness in this sense may not just be restricted to the field of kinship but may refer to the field of ethnicity and 'race' too. If procreation beliefs tell you who you are, they equally tell you who you are not, and in this paper I shall examine how procreation beliefs illuminate the understanding of ethnic and racial difference in the central Andes of South America.

The Andes are home to a number of indigenous groups who can be variously grouped and the study of ethnicity in the Andes and highland South America has a rich history. It is by now received wisdom among Andean scholars that the distinction between indians[1] and non-indians is fluid, historically contingent and arbitrary. How this mutable distinction is constituted is, however, a matter for considerable debate. Many writers on the

Andes see these differences as based on a mixture of ethnicity and class (see for example van den Berghe and Primov 1977; Gose 1994) whereas others focus their attention much more closely on cultural practices and beliefs (Skar 1982; Allen 1988). More recently Mary Weismantel (1997) has called upon scholars to re-examine the notion of 'race' in the Andean context and in this vein, for example, Ben Orlove (1998) has illustrated how the racial difference between indians and non-indians in Peru is rooted in differing relations to earth. But earth here is mainly a trope for discussing social difference: indians' adobe houses and earthernware pots, their proximity to the earth, these are emblems of difference, not its roots, which must surely lie elsewhere. By the same token, it does not follow from Weismantel's argument (1997) that just because one can identify pervasive racism in the Andes, the differences which produce the negative stereotyping are usefully examined under the category 'race'. Moreover, race can be defined so broadly as to render it a very blunt analytical instrument.

A very different approach is one taken by Catherine Allen (1988) who finds difference created and sustained in communal beliefs, most specifically the chewing of coca. Allen's approach is useful in that it looks beyond categories of class and ethnicity and begins to consider how practices (such as coca-chewing) and the meanings imputed to these practices constitute difference. Difference is rooted in practice and in this sense it is performative. It is not, however, altogether clear why or how these practices actually produce different kinds of people, that is, what it is about chewing coca that creates a different order of being from non-coca-chewers.

A number of scholars (e.g. Isbell 1978:73; Allen 1988) have noted that indians themselves have an understanding of difference based around the categories *jaqi* (Aymara), *runa* (Quechua) which mean simply 'people', and *q'ara* in both languages (variably *qala*), which literally means 'peeled' or 'bare' and can be glossed as someone bereft of essential culture. For the people of Pocobaya[2] where my fieldwork was conducted a very similar understanding is evident: *q'aras* are those who are not part of a community. A community is a corporate unit where people hold land in common but, more importantly, a community is seen in terms of reciprocal aid between people and also a relationship of reciprocity with the tellurian spirits. What makes people people, then, is not outward appearance or descent from a particular group in history but a particular kind of relationship with other people and earth spirits. At the very root of the *jaqi/q'ara* distinction for Pocobayenos are not historical events or biological notions of difference but the processes which create fully constituted people; these processes, moreover, are not rooted in physiology but in social and ritual practice. It is important to note here that relatedness is primarily based, not on an idea of shared substance as is the case with many of the examples in this volume, but on a set of relationships marked by ritual and practice rather in the manner in which Allen (1988) describes difference in terms of coca.

This is not to say that substance is never the focus of difference in the Andes. Indeed, one of the arguments I make below is that fat and its regulated flow between the human and spirit world is part of what constitutes the difference between *jaqi* and *q'ara*. However, to focus solely on the substance as if it emblematized difference and ignore the relational and performative aspects which make it meaningful would be to conspire in reducing the difference between indians and non-indians to one of race. Similarly, although looking at icons of difference such as earth and coca sheds much light on how difference is articulated, there are limits to this analysis for it only tells us so much about the nature of a person. One needs to look then at how personhood is understood, how persons come into being and how these might be different to other kinds of people. If procreation 'concerns beliefs about where, from what, and how a person comes into being' (Delaney 1991:147) then examining procreation beliefs may shed a great deal of light on how people understand differences.

'How a person comes into being' is not however the same as how humans are born. Persons are not simply born but are created over time. The direct translation into Aymara of 'to create a person' would be *jaqichasiña,* a term which in Pocobaya is most commonly used for 'marriage'. This suggests at least that personhood is not something conceived or conferred until well into adulthood and, moreover, that it is a lengthy process. In this paper I shall concentrate on the first few years of life which mark the development of personhood, although it will be clear that this is a process that continues into adulthood and beyond. Underlying this process of maturation are the concepts which relate the person to the moral communities of the human and spirit worlds. In brief, many of the rituals and concepts of maturation explicitly relate these two communities to each other. If these rituals and relationships create a kind of person they also exclude another kind of person. Thus procreation beliefs, beliefs relating to how persons are created, illuminate greatly the difference between indians and non-indians for the people of Pocobaya and other similar groups.

First, though, I would like to make a brief sketch of Pocobaya and its social and physical geography.

POCOBAYA

Pocobaya is a hamlet of 220 people in the Bolivian Andes. The people are Aymara-speakers and are agriculturists who benefit from the sharp relief of the Andes to exploit a number of different ecological zones. Pocobayenos are fortunate in that their lands go high enough to produce potatoes and low enough to produce wheat and maize, but with increasing erosion and population the land of Pocobaya is insufficient to meet the needs of all the people who live on it. Seasonal wage migration is therefore a necessity for most men. Despite this, Pocobayenos, as other indigenous agriculturists, are very much focused on the land. Even people who have more or less permanently moved from the village return to sow and harvest their land and thus maintain membership of the community. This provides them with little economic benefit but is clearly an important part of an identity they wish to maintain (cf. Albó et al. 1987). To rupture this relationship with the land and the community through permanent migration is to effect a radical change in identity, from being a *jaqi* to being a *q'ara*. In national terms being an indian primarily means living on the land in such a community. The move away from the land to the cities or mines changes one's ethnic status to that of a *cholo*, an urbanized indian and eventually, with upward mobility and a good ability in Spanish, to a *mestizo* a person of mixed race or culture.[3] The distinction between being an indian (*indio)* and a member of the large and predominant *mestizo* community is highly significant in the Bolivian context. It is the difference between being a member of a marginalized, relatively powerless and frequently disdained group and being part of the metropolitan culture. Being an indian does have some advantages, however, namely being part of a strong and supportive community without which life on a highland smallholding would be virtually impossible. As I have noted elsewhere (Canessa 1993), virtually all ritual life in Pocobaya in one way or another deals with either the community of the living or the community of spirits on which the human community depends. Given that the community is so important in one's life one might suspect that birth into the community would be a highly celebrated event. In fact, although births are noted by the community, they are not marked by any public ritual or celebration. This is quite in contrast to all other 'life crisis' events in Pocobaya and underlines the fact that one is not born into the community but, rather, one has to be received into it. Nor is one born into a descent group since, unlike in other parts of the Bolivian Andes (e.g. Arnold 1989; Abercrombie 1998), there are no descent groups in Pocobaya so birth does not even confer membership to such a group.

Personhood is a process. It is not rooted in the simple fact of being born or in shared substance, but in one's action upon the world. In very much a similar way, gender is based on activity and relationship rather than physiological difference (Canessa 1997). In this manner, difference between indians and non-indians is not reducible from an emic perspective to a basic shared substance or even shared descent,[4] but is something rooted in the practice of life, in production and agency.

Agency is at all levels underwritten by the spirits to whom offerings must be regularly made. The successful running of the household is at the centre of adults' lives and one aspect of this, of course, is producing children. Producing a large number of children is not, however, desirable and people are keen to limit their families to reasonable proportions. People are very aware that large numbers of children will only make them poorer in the long-term as well as the short term: a large family is difficult to feed and there simply is not enough land for all to inherit. This perhaps partly accounts for the reasons why births are not as celebrated as in other cultures where more children mean more wealth or more members of the lineage. In Pocobaya the ability to produce children is an indication that the married couple can productively maintain a household and reproduce; for the child, birth merely produces the raw material out of which a person may be created.

CONCEPTION AND BIRTH

Fiestas are the points in the annual calendar by which both conceptions and births are reckoned. The annual cycle in Pocobaya is marked by periods of sociality and periods when people interact very little beyond the household. Throughout most of the year people confine themselves to their household units and occasionally work together with close kin. There is little social contact with other households; there is not, for example, a custom of generalized visiting. Fiestas are, however, a time of intense sociality: agricultural work ceases and all the adults of the community will eat and drink together, sometimes for several days. This is a time of heightened sensitivity: people cry, laugh, shout, fight and flirt with great intensity. It is also a time for engaging with the nature spirits, either through direct offerings or more generally through the community celebrating together. The sharing of alcohol is a way of communicating with the spirits (Saignes 1993) as is chewing coca leaves (*akult'asiña*) (Allen 1988:137 ff.). It is thus through fiestas that the community spirit and solidarity are re-created and affirmed. The tension between household and community (cf. Albó 1975) is submerged in fiestas and the whole community shares food and drink as if they were one household.[5]

Fiestas are also a time when people are eroticized. Dancing, for example, is said to increase erotic awareness in adults as its function is to encourage the earth goddess's fertility by sexually stimulating her. One reason then why conceptions are reckoned in terms of fiestas is that people are more sexually aroused during this period and several Pocobayenos commented to me that this was also a time of greater sexual activity.[6]

Fiesta time is also the time when young couples typically choose to elope. Young couples may very well have initiated a sexual relationship long before and this relationship may indeed be known if not acknowledged by both sets of parents, but the first stage in a marriage is when a young man 'abducts' a young woman and takes her to his parents' house where they spend the night. If a young woman or girl were to become pregnant before this event it would be very difficult to persuade the potential father to support her, but once the relationship is made public in this way he would be considered responsible for the maintenance of any offspring.

Conception occurs with the union of semen and menstrual blood (*jatha wilampi juntasiya*). As a result, some Pocobayenos stated that conception is easiest during menstruation, a belief shared by people in the Aymara-speaking communities of Qaqachaka (Arnold 1989:202 ff; Arnold and Yapita 1996). This is, however, by no means necessary and it is known that a woman who menstruates irregularly or even not at all may still conceive. Menstruation is known as *wila phaxsi*, the monthly blood, but despite this many women from Pocobaya do not menstruate regularly. This is most likely due to long periods of lactation, frequent pregnancies and poor nutrition.

Despite the fact that the man and woman contribute to the creation of the foetus, there is no sense that semen and blood contribute to certain parts such as blood and bones (cf. Bloch 1992) or that in conception blood lines and semen lines are intermingling (c.f. Arnold 1989), as indeed we might suspect, given that there is no meaningful sense of 'lineage' in Pocobaya. Without such corporate units or matrilateral and patrilateral kin recognized in a distinguishable way, ideas surrounding conception quite simply reflect the belief that men and women create children together.

Blood and semen combine to create a growing, formless, bloody mass (*wila muruqu*) until the fourth month of gestation when the foetus begins to move. At this point the foetus will have hair and bones and becomes known as a foetus or *sullu*.

Throughout the pregnancy the couple will make regular offerings to the condor-falcon (*kunturmamani*) who is the principal household god.[7] This is especially important should the woman become sick during pregnancy. Offerings made to the *kunturmamani* will ensure that her spirit (*ajayu*) returns and the pregnancy proceeds to its full course.

During pregnancy, the woman will continue her chores but they will gradually diminish, particularly the heavy ones, as the pregnancy develops. A pregnant mother has recourse to three specialists in case there are any problems during her pregnancy: the *yatiri,* the *qulliri* and the *uswiri.* The *yatiri* deals with problems of a spiritual nature, those matters that involve the *ajayu* (soul). The *qulliri* deals with more superficial illnesses, those that involve *chuyma*, the life force, and the *uswiri* is best described as a midwife.[8] The *uswiri* is also a *qulliri* but specializes in the problems of pregnancy. She will massage the abdomen and predict the date of the birth. This date is the date of the fiesta during which the *uswiri* believes the child will be born. She will also make sure the foetus is positioned properly by performing *thalthapiña* – having the mother lie on an *awayu* (carrying cloth) and manoeuvring the *awayu* by the ends.

None of these specialists is present at the actual birth unless there is a particular problem. A birth is very much a private, household affair, and not much attention is accorded it by villagers beyond those directly involved. It generally takes place at home where the mother-to-be is attended by her husband. This is in sharp contrast to the people of Kaata studied by Bastien to whom 'delivery is a female activity from which men are excluded' (Bastien 1978:87). In Pocobaya it is the man's duty to make sure the woman is comfortable, warm and well-fed. He will fill the room with smoke as this is thought to assist the birth. The mother is fed on lamb broth during labour and for several days after the birth, as well as other rich and fortifying foods.

Once the child is born it is cleaned and swaddled but not fed until at least twenty-four hours after birth; in some areas I was told the baby is not fed for three days. The reason given is that this makes the baby hardy but it may also be the case that a very weak baby will die quickly and thus not tax the emotional and economic resources of the family.[9]

I was given two differing accounts regarding the disposal of the afterbirth (*parisa*). I was told it is buried either inside the house or by a brook with fast-flowing water. Dark areas of houses (especially corners) as well as brooks are associated with the tellurian spirits. It appears that the afterbirth, metonymically linked to the child, must be held in the bosom of the tellurian spirits and protected from damaging sunlight. If the afterbirth is not buried by the brook, I was told, the baby's face is believed to become deformed and it may lead to death. The child itself is vulnerable to light and great care is taken not to expose its face to sunlight.[10] A child, as every living thing, is the product of the power of the *Pachamama*, the chthonic earth mother. In the first days of life especially, it must be protected from the inimical forces of the upper world, especially the sun, which is its presiding deity. The consequences for the mother of not burying the afterbirth are severe and may lead to her death. This is perhaps a recognition of the very high danger she is in herself and generally people are much more concerned for the mother's health than the new-born.

NAMING

Sutiyaña,[11] naming, is the first ritual which acknowledges a child's identity as separate from its mother's. This small ceremony is attended by the immediate family and usually, in Pocobaya, by the catechist who will baptize the child.

Salt and water are mixed into a paste resembling fat (*lik'ja-mawa*) and then daubed on the baby's mouth. Salt is considered to be a defining attribute of civilized humans (cf. Harris 1980) and through this ritual the child enters the civilized world. Body fat, which the paste of salt and water is said to resemble, is believed to be a source of essential life force (*chuyma*), with the diminution or loss of it entailing illness or death, and fat (*lik'i*) is a common offering to the spirits as a substitute for human sacrifice (cf. Bastien 1978; Sallnow 1987).

In the *sutiyaña,* however, the 'fat' is not animal or human fat but salt and what is enacted is not an offering to the spirits but an anointment of the child. Through this ritual the child receives its essential humanity from the underworld but this creates a debt. In exchange for the ability to act productively upon the world the spirits must be offered fat in return. This may be in the form of animal fat but ultimately the debt can only be repaid by the return of the human body into the earth whence it came.

The *sutiyaña* marks the beginning of a relationship with the spirits and with the human community. The substance of fat marks the difference between those who engage with the spirits and those who do not. Indeed, non-indians are believed to steal fat through their nefarious agents known as *kharisiris*. This powerful expression of the fear of racial violence (Weismantel 1997) does not, however, mean that we have located the substance of racial difference in the Andes for difference is not so much rooted in the substance of fat (since, after all, it can be acquired by 'racial others', if illegitimately), but in the human and extra-human relationships it articulates.

These extra-human relationships initiated by the *sutiyaña* are not solely confined to the sphere of chthonic spirits since the child also receives a Christian baptism. If the child dies before this simple ceremony, it is not buried in the cemetery, but far away from the village in a barren place called Kimurpata. After establishing its relationship with the chthonic spirits, the child is anointed in a ritual that makes it a Christian (*kristyanu*). Baptism is important to the child for, apart from its relationship with the spirits of below residing in the *Manqhapacha*, it must also live in a world where other forces dominate. In a Christian age, not to be a Christian leaves one vulnerable to the powers of a hostile god. The combined ceremony, then, establishes a connection with the source of life and humanity on the one hand whilst underwriting it with a rite of inclusion into the world of the presiding deity.[12]

If the child dies before the *sutiyaña*, at this stage of its existence it is considered totally unsocialized and in a sense non-human, for it has neither speech nor even a name. An unnamed baby is considered to be still a foetus (*sullu*) and it is for this reason that data on neonatal deaths are so difficult to obtain. It is impossible to know if one is recording infanticide or neonatal deaths and with time a mother will tend not to consider neonatal deaths as births at all. On several occasions when talking to women about the number of babies they had had, they omitted births of babies that died in the first weeks or even months of life, of which I happened to be aware. It is during the period before the salt ceremony that infanticide, when it does occur, is most likely to take place.[13]

The new-born's status as foetus clearly indicates that birth in itself does not produce persons even if it does provide some of the raw materials. It is not until the first rituals that a foetus (*sullu*) becomes a baby (*wawa*).

A child's *ajayu* (spirit), even after it has been baptized, is not considered to be secure in the body and is particularly vulnerable to *sustu* (Sp. *susto*, fright) where the *ajayu* leaves the body due to some kind of shock or fright.[14] Punishing a child too severely, I was told, can effect *sustu* and loss of the *ajayu*. The *ajayu* gradually becomes more firmly entrenched as the child grows up into adolescence although adults, too, can suffer from the loss of the *ajayu* due to fright or shock. It may very well be that the belief that *sustu* is particularly prevalent in children is a way of rationalizing high child mortality which is articulated in terms of the process of the socialization of the child: that is, there is a correlation between the children's decreasing mortality and the process by which the community invests the child with more and more status and affection.

Swaddling is an important part of how a child is protected for it is a way of containing the child. The baby is incontinent on a number of levels: it has no control over its bodily functions but also its spirit (*ajayu*) is not properly contained and is easily lost, thus the high rate of childhood death. A child is tightly bound with several cloths and the final item is a bright and colourful woven cloth called a *wak'a*. The *wak'a* is woven by the child's mother and is believed to protect the child against spirit loss. In other parts of the contemporary Andes *wak'as* are mountain deities and in the Incaic and colonial periods the word was used to describe a much wider range of deities. In Pocobaya '*wak'a*' is only used for this cloth but its function is clearly one that would lend to associations with the ancestral spirits.

As time goes by, the baby will be swaddled for less and less time. The mother will carry the baby in her *awayu* carrying cloth and breastfeed on demand until the child is about six months old, when the weaning process begins with some weak coffee. Nevertheless the child will continue breastfeeding to the end of the second year although, of course, less frequently. Full weaning tends to occur earlier if the mother becomes pregnant once again.

In a large family the principal care of the child is taken by one of the daughters. It will be her responsibility to carry the baby in the *awayu,* comforting it when it cries. If the baby needs milk she will take it to the mother. In general a child's parents will pay little attention to it; its siblings will generally play with it and, quite importantly, teach it to speak. Older siblings will teach their younger brothers and sisters to speak by getting them to repeat words, and they often make it into some sort of game.

It is typically the case that not much physical affection is directed towards children. In fact, it is safe to say that children are largely ignored beyond their most vital requirements. In Pocobaya a baby will very rarely be referred to by name, the generic *wawa* (baby) being much more common. It is generally not until a child is old enough to walk and talk and perform tasks that it will actually be called by name. Spedding notes that for Aymara-speakers of the *yungas* (warm valleys) a child's name is generally first used when a parent or sibling wishes it to fetch or do something, that is, in an imperative (1989:292).

It has been argued (e.g. Kurtz 1992) that such child-rearing practices and the absence of 'mirroring' on the part of the parent with the child allow for a different development of a personal identity: the child, finding that its personality is not affirmed as an individual, seeks a personality in the group.[15] Whether it is because of such child-rearing practices or not, it is very clear that Pocobayenos have little sense of the bounded individual as has developed in the West. Personhood in Pocobaya is more accurately described in terms of social rather than individual personalities; it is not so much that people are divisible into substantially different relationships but that they enter into a contained web of relationships. The containment of this web is important for, even though Pocobayenos do have relationships outside the community, identity is very much rooted in the community. This was most clearly outlined to me when I first arrived in Pocobaya. I was taken to a high point with a good view and my companion, Edmundo, explained the surrounding social geography to me: all the visible villages were populated by murderers and thieves; Pocobaya was the only place where good people resided. This was despite the fact that many Pocobayenos, of course, have relatives in all these villages.

RITUCHA

The point at which the child is first publicly recognized by this moral community as a member is in the *ritucha* or first haircutting. The *ritucha*, an Andean-wide rite (cf. Bastien 1978; Carter and Mamani 1982; Allen 1988), marks the entry of a child into the world as a social person. Until the *ritucha* the child's hair has been neither cut nor washed and through the ritual the child goes from a wild, dirty and unkempt state to a social one. Another word for *ritucha* is *muruña* which also means cutting off a bull's horns. In the same way as a bull is rendered tame by removing its horns, the 'wild' child is socialized by removing its unkempt hair.

Speech is an important element in the distinction between the wild and the social, human and non-human (Harris 1980) and the *ritucha* takes place when a child has begun to speak. The socializing element of the ritual is underlined by the fact that, unlike the naming ceremony, the entire community is invited. In this way the child is introduced as a social being to the community and vice versa: the *ritucha* marks the 'social' birth of the child as distinct from its physical birth.[16]

The ceremony begins with a libation to the spirit of the house, the *kunturmamani*, who has watched over the woman and her foetus during the pregnancy. The *pärinu* and *märina* (godfather and godmother) will start cutting the child's matted locks and they put money in an *inkuña*, a woven cloth used for offerings made from llama wool. They are then followed by all the adults present. The *inkuña* is a cloth used for ritual purposes such as coca divination and its inclusion here marks the child as a ritually significant being. This is the child's *inkuña* and when all the locks of hair are collected they are wrapped in the *inkuña* and stored in the rafters of the house. This is an offering to the *kunturmamani* in order that s/he may be honoured and, in turn, cast a watchful eye over the child.

The ceremony ends with joint thanks given to the *kunturmamani* and other spirits and then the party celebrates with food, alcohol and coca. The sharing of food, alcohol and coca also has a ritual value, for it is through such activities that people engage with the chthonic spirits who will vicariously consume with the celebrating community. The hair-cutting ceremony is the first ritual through which the child is formally introduced to the community. It also marks the transition from infancy (*wawa*) to becoming a boy or girl (*yuqalla* or *imilla*, respectively). After this point the child may officially be mourned at death and during *Todos Santos*, the Feast of the Dead, s/he may be remembered at the grave through the presentation of favourite foods as is the case with deceased adults. Even so, it is rare for a child to be mourned in this way and it is almost exclusively adults who are remembered in *Todos Santos*. The first hair-cutting also marks the beginning of the age of responsibility and from this age on the child is said to begin with household chores. The reality is, however, that a couple of years pass before the child begins to make a significant contribution to the household. The point, though, is that the child is deemed capable of productive labour and the ability to act upon the world productively is an ability that is deemed to come ultimately from the mountain spirits.

Related to this is the importance of labour in creating and defining human beings. A person is not someone who simply is but someone who does; that is, personhood is performative. A gendered person is someone who performs the tasks appropriate to a particular gender and only secondarily a person of a particular biological sex. Thus a child does not become a social person until s/he is capable of performing certain tasks. This ability is accorded by the community and the earth spirits, who first publicly recognize the child at the *ritucha* ceremony. The child moves from a semi-wild state with dirty, matted locks in which it is not even a named person, to a human being, recognized and anointed by the community and capable of productive action.

Of course, a child at this age is capable of fairly limited productive action and the *ritucha* really only marks one stage in the acquisition of personhood. Childhood and adolescence are still marked by considerable social ambiguity. At an early age and throughout adolescence children will be given the task of herding animals. Leaving early in the morning and returning late in the evening, they will spend day after day far away from the village under the burning sun or cold rain. There they will join their peers with whom they will spend the day but it is a sociality far removed from the adult world. When the adults are enjoying themselves in fiestas or engaged in other communal ritual events such as funerals and wakes they are still often obliged to herd the animals. Even when they do attend it is on the periphery of action: they will not share food, alcohol and coca leaves with their peers as their parents do; nor will they be allowed to address community meetings or have a say in decisions.

It is not until marriage that one is a fully constituted person as suggested by the term for marriage: *jaqichasiña*, to make a person. As a married person one begins to assume some of the many community offices, to be asked to be a godparent, to inherit land, exchange labour and start a household. As a married adult one also makes regular offerings to the spirits of the land and household. As we saw above, the assumption of communal offices and the exchange of labour are among the things which distinguish indians from non-indians. One can also add the sharing of coca and alcohol as well as a ritual orientation. All of these are testaments to a relationship between individuals and their community and the community with the spirits.

One of the more important aspects of this integration is the establishment of a series of reciprocal relationships. This kind of relationship, paradigmatically an exchange of labour, has been described by many researchers as being one of the fundamental differences between true 'people' and others, for unlike those with other *jaqi,* exchanges with urban-dwellers are described as being asymmetrical and often highly exploitative (see Mayer 1975; ; Isbell 1978; Allen 1988:93 among others). This kind of relationship is not confined to the human world, for relationships with the spirit world are also so conceived and this accounts for the intimacy of the relationship Pocobayenos have with these spirits. As we saw above, one important aspect of this exchange is the anointment by fat (as salt) and the life-long relationship which entails regular offerings of fat in various forms.

This process continues at death and beyond. After death a person is remembered for three years by name after which s/he is properly remembered as part of the collectivity of spirits which are the moral guardians of the community and provide rain for crops (Harris 1982). In this way personhood in Pocobaya is the gradual integration of the individual into the community to the point where the individual merges into the apotheosis of the community – the spirit world. As personhood develops the arbitrariness of birth, the power of sex, the finality of death are controlled, anointed and integrated into communal structures. Personhood develops to its highest point when individuality is extinguished.

CONCLUSION: MAKING PERSONS, MARKING DIFFERENCE

Following Delaney's (1991) insight that ideas surrounding birth are not merely reflective of more generalized ideas of where humans are in the world but are constitutive of such relationships, we can see that Pocobayeno ideas surrounding birth are part of a more generalized understanding of how human beings relate to the land, the members of their community and the world beyond.

As I mentioned above, what makes a person a person is one's relationship with land and community but not just any land and any community. The land on which someone lives and works is a very personalized land with which people have quite intimate relationships. As Michael Sallnow has noted, as people move through the landscape they experience it kinaesthetically (1987) and, in common with other parts of the Andes, Pocobayenos have a plethora of toponyms for virtually every outcrop of rock and turn in the stream, and these names are given by the ancestors, the *achachilas*. But as we have seen, in a profound sense, Pocobayenos are of the land and to leave it is, for many, a most traumatic process for it changes entirely their conception of themselves.

There are, at the same time, strong social and economic forces impelling Pocobayenos to leave, not least of which is the fact that the land can no longer support the entire community. As is true of many migrants, some leave with every intention of returning but never quite make it home. Even the successful migrant may have very conflicting feelings about leaving the land and community. One such person who became quite wealthy in the gold mines occasionally returned drunk and maudlin and stayed in the village for a few days. He would cry and apologize to all for his behaviour, for abandoning the community, for abandoning the land. After a few days' work in the fields, shedding his boots for sandals so he could feel the earth, he would return to his interests in the capital or his mine until his next visit.

But it should also be clear why migration has such a profound effect on ethnicity. If personal identity as I have described it is so rooted in place and community and the relations of these to agricultural activity, living in an urban setting without the streams and the mountains, let alone the fields and crops, one's sense of person must inevitably be different. It appears then that 'indianness' is so bound up in a particular lifestyle, both from the emic and etic perspective, that it does not easily survive the move to the city (Harris 1995). This is the paradox facing those intellectuals who seek an Aymara national identity. They can address the educated and urbanized migrants in terms of flags and nationhood, a language which is clearly European, but these ideas have no resonance among those whose sense of identity is founded on entirely different precepts, not on nationhood or descent, but particular practices and relationships and, above all, a different sense of what constitutes *jaqi*, a person.

The Andes provide a historical and cultural context in which social difference is not easily reduced to class, ethnicity or race. These modes of analysis are, of course, highly valuable but they tend to be reductive rather than dynamic; they do, moreover, tend to an etic rather than emic perspective. Through an examination of procreation beliefs in the village of Pocobaya I hope to have shed some light on how difference is conceived, created and sustained from an emic perspective. Identity is shown to be an active process rather than a state, a process which is sustained over a lifetime of human and extra-human relationships. This analysis goes beyond trying to identify the substance of racial difference; it avoids the quandaries of people in the same formal class position having a different ethnic identity, and obviates the problems of locating ethnicity in particular cultural forms such as language and dress. An examination of procreation beliefs can thus be highly illuminating in examining how people distinguish themselves from others, because at the root of all such differentiation are differing conceptions of what properly constitutes a person.

NOTES

A version of this paper was first delivered at the 'Procreation' conference organized by Peter Loizos at the LSE in the summer of 1996. I am grateful to him and the other participants for the general stimulating discussion and specific comments on the paper.

1 The term 'indian' is obviously one of European origin and in its American usage denoted a simple power relationship, the difference between conqueror and conquered. Over the past centuries, although the status of the 'indian' as well as the way that identity has been understood has changed, it has always denoted a difference in status and power and, moreover, it has been non-indians who have decided who is and is not an 'indian'. In this paper 'indian' is used principally when talking from an external perspective. Although those denominated as 'indians' have this identity imposed upon them, the manner in which they understand this identity is very different. When talking about this internal perspective, I shall use the term *jaqi*.

I prefer the term 'indian' over 'indigenous'. 'Indigenous' is drawn from natural history and means 'belonging naturally to the region'. There is a certain absurdity in talking of indigeneity in the Andes since the vast majority of Andeans have some descent from the people the conquistadors met. Indigenous also implies being of 'pure' native descent. One would need to include millions of such people who do not see themselves as indigenous but are seen by others as indigenous and thus the term has limited analytical purchase. 'Indian' on the other hand, in the American context, more clearly indicates a culturally constructed identity. In the American context, 'indian' is an ethnic, not national term and therefore I follow the usage of writing this word in lower case in the same way as other such categories, e.g. *mestizo*, black, mulatto (see Wade 1997:121).

2 Fieldwork was conducted between 1989 and 1992 and again in 1993 and 1998.

3 A mestizo originally referred to a person of 'mixed race'. In the contemporary Andes, however, being a *mestizo* has much more to do with place or residence, occupation, dress and fluency in Spanish than any putatively mixed ancestry.

4 It is, however, true that it is considered important to engage with the autochthonous spirits and that one is considered 'of' these spirits, but this is not the same as simply asserting descent from original inhabitants.

5 It is also the case that many tensions surface during fiestas, assisted no doubt by alcohol. As people are sleep-deprived and drunk these tensions arise, often violently, but they are also quickly resolved and I have argued (1993) that this has a cathartic effect, preventing disputes and rivalries mouldering indefinitely.

6 I was told by some informants that if conception occurs when one or both of the couple are drunk a miscarriage or malformation occurs. Others, however, denied the significance of sobriety in conception. A distinction is made between the sex acts of adolescents which occasionally occur when they are herding and those of adults. Adolescent sex is considered 'wild' because the adolescents are unmarried and is performed beyond the community boundaries (cf. Harris 1980:77). These acts are not so much immoral as valueless since they occur between people who are socially immature, and therefore do not possess sufficient agency, and in a place far from the community.

7 Both the condor and falcon are associated with the mountain ancestors, especially when they act as messengers.

8 The word *uswiri* comes from *usu*, pregnant (it also means illness), and the suffix *iri* which indicates profession.

9 By my calculations the child mortality in Pocobaya (that is, up to five years of age) is 26 per cent. The figure may actually be higher as neonatal deaths (within the first week) are almost never recorded or considered as a live birth. This figure was obtained at by comparing household birth and death rates for the previous five years. There is almost certainly under-reporting the number of births as well as deaths, especially the deaths of neonates. In a number of cases there was a dispute in the family as to how many children had been born. Although I attempted to account for this, the figure of 26 per cent must be taken as a conservative estimate. This figure is, however, comparable to data collected by nurses and doctors working in rural highland Bolivia, although one must presume they face similar problems in counting.

10 Darkness is naturally associated with the underworld (*Manqhapacha*) spirits and light with the upper-world (*Alaxpacha*) spirits presided over by the Christian God and his son/sun. The two spheres are often seen as being inimical to one another. The sun is associated with the Christian God with whom Pocobayenos do not have the same kind of relationship as with other deities. The principal way in which the Christian God affects the lives of Pocobayenos is by bringing hail. This God is generally a punishing God and I learned of no instances when he had a benevolent or productive effect on people's lives.

11 *Suti.ya.ña*: *suti*, name; *ya*, verbal suffix, 'to make or do'; *ña*, infinitive. Thus: to name.

12 Possession of a baptismal certificate, moreover, is the easiest way of obtaining a Bolivian identity card and, in practice, the only way open to indians.

13 The most common method, I was told, is to place the baby out in the cold at night where the cold mountain air usually has the desired effect by morning. Data on infanticide are difficult to obtain, but as

far as I can gather infanticide occurs when the baby has a physical defect or if it appears quite sick. Unwanted pregnancies are usually dealt with by recourse to herbal abortifacients or by a visit to the pharmacist in the nearest market town.

14 Once when I was travelling past a remote hamlet in the cordillera, I was seen by several children who ran away frightened. Their father caught up with me and demanded compensation for the *sustu* I had caused for they would surely now become sick.

15 I would not wish to impute a simple causal relationship to child-rearing practices and strong group identity, but the intensely communal nature of Aymara personal identity has been noted by others (cf. Albó 1985) and early child-rearing practices may very well be the first step in the creation of such an identity.

16 Bloch and Guggenheim's (1981) observation that baptism implies that biological birth is insufficient to create a 'proper' human being holds equally well for the *ritucha*. It is clear that a baby born without any ritual is considered something less than a person in any sense.

CHAPTER 5

EVERY INFANT IS BORN WITH ITS 'YOUNGER SIBLING'

CHILDBIRTH AND CARE AMONG AMURANG FISHERMEN

SINI CEDERCREUTZ

This paper outlines how a fisherman's child and its 'younger sibling' (placenta) enter the world in the central coastal villages of Amurang, North Sulawesi.[1] Amurang consists of a collection of villages, many dependent on fishing, with a high concentration of schools, churches and government offices, as it is a sub-district capital, in Minahasa. Amurang childbirth and caring arrangements are, indisputably, domains of central importance to the local people. They involve many cherished beliefs and practices which represent the local religious and medical pluralism: Amurang fishermen's Protestant Christianity (*agama kristen protestan*) lives a contested and continuously renegotiated coexistence with the 'teachings of our forefathers'. The latter is a non-codified body of practical and esoteric knowledge, increasingly labelled as the 'religion of yesterday' (*agama dulu*). Part of it is the 'tradition of the sea' (*tradisi lao*) of the *giop*-sailing fishermen, most of whom are Borgo people (*orang borgo*) with European surnames. These beliefs remain largely hidden and absent from the official, 'modern' Indonesian discourse aimed at outsiders, for reasons that are beyond the scope of this paper. All Minahasans, fishermen included, are concerned that they do not appear as uncivilized indigenes practising polytheist worship of ancestors, outlawed by the state ideology (Pancasila) which is part of the Preamble to the Constitution. They see themselves as an important pious and educated religious minority in the world's most populous Muslim country. Both western bio-medical health care and the national Indonesian school curricula have made inroads into local practices. Among Amurang Borgo fishermen, the supra-local concepts of illness actiology, relatedness and ideas of the model family are readily agreed upon but less often in evidence within midwifery, caring for children, or in private family planning.

A traditional midwife (*dukun bayi*) and another former traditional midwife, who had undergone a short medical course run by government health extension worker and is now called *mama biang* (*I. bidan*) allowed me to join them on their visits to see pre- and post-natal women, and to women with fertility problems. These elderly and respected widows clarified for me their concepts and practices concerning procreation, pregancy and childbirth. Whereas Javanese *bidan* are usually the younger midwives who work at health centres (*Puskesmas*)[2] and accompany the elder *dukun*,[3] there is no such difference in Amurang where the *dukun* and *mama biang* operate separately, from their homes, and originally entered the profession by following the example of their mothers.

Both the prospective parents and the midwife can take various steps to protect the health of the infant. Under the auspices of the experienced midwives with 'good' (*bagus*) and 'cool hands' (*tangan dingin*), the union of material and immaterial substances in the form of an infant is a joint product of its parents, the ancestors and God. New-born children are prone to die in Amurang, but even for those who survive physical birth, the process of becoming a person remains incomplete for some time. These issues of personhood and health offer fascinating insights into Amurang perceptions of the conceptualization of illness and health.

The long process of cooperation between an Amurang fish-wife and a midwife begins at the moment when a woman has difficulties in conceiving, and hopefully ends in a succesfully completed labour. Midwives are women's collaborators until some time after the birth. The ensuing burial of the afterbirth and the conversion of the remains of the infant's umbilical cord into 'medicine' (*obat*) are conceptually part of what it means to give birth. At this point, the intimate relationship between the two women is terminated, and debts are paid in kind and money. Midwives' knowledge of the local 'medicines of the land' and their massaging and other healing skills are greatly appreciated by fishermen. Their meagre economies would be upset if they had to pay the local health centre's charges, or those of the local Protestant hospital.

Childbirth is a process of considerable length and involves notions of unselfish care and indebtedness on behalf of all the actors involved; childbirth practices tell about the local meanings and the importance of children. This paper concludes by widening this focus onto the role of 'mutual nurturance' (*baku-piara*) and of mutual love/pity (*bakusayang*) between cohabiting spouses. These are also salient idioms about how parental responsibilities establish the status of children, whether these are born in or outside wedlock, have been temporarily borrowed or adopted. In other words, the local notions of midwifery, infant treatment and childcare make explicit the cultural and social framework within which they operate.

APPROACHING AMURANG

Approached from the sea against the rugged volcanoes, Amurang appears first as white stucco-decorated church towers in a dense forest of coconut trees. The twelve motorized sailing ships (*giop*) are outnumbered by hundreds of outrigger canoes. Whether *giop* men return from their travels after fish within a day or after several months, their wives continue to manage households and to work as fish curers and sellers. By the standards of local agriculturalists, most Borgo fishermen are poor. Farmers and administrators judge fishermen to be lazy, uncivilized and uninterested in planning for tomorrow, failing to recognize the basic limitations of the economies of scale in traditional[4] fishing: landlessness, seasonality, the unpredictability of the marine environment and the market, and their strategy of the minimizing risks rather than maximizing profits.

It was indeed the case also a hundred years ago that 'all the roads and fish meet in Amurang'. Like other major Minahasan coastal ports which were Dutch garrison towns, there were Chinese, Arab, Malay and Eurasian traders and travellers, and Dutch officials. There were the 'Indo-Europeans', or Eurasians, who were descendants of inter-ethnic marriages between the admired Europeans and the indigenes. Those acknowledged by their European fathers came under the European law. Even as early as 1758, others were legally designated as an in-between category and brought over to Minahasa by the Dutch from the 'Spice islands', mainly the north and central Moluccas (Watuseke 1968:30–1, 51–2; Watuseke and Henley 1994:365). In Dutch they were called *inlandse burgers*, native citizens or, in the local rendering the Borgo people. They were a class of people higher in status than the indigenes but lower than their overlords, first the Dutch East Indies Company (VOC), later the Batavian colonial government under the crown of the Netherlands (Graafland [1869]1991:472–5; Bakhuitzen van den Brink [1880]1915). The Borgo people had to accept baptism and become Christian. They took European surnames: Dutch, Flemish or German names like Ottay, Heydemans, Peters, Stahl or Durandt.[5] They traded their special legal status and corvée exemptions for armed peace-keeping duties on land and for the protection of Dutch trade interests against the pirates at sea. They were obligted to live in the *burger* quarters and in theory could not buy land (Kristanto 1995; DepDikBud 1992). For their food, they turned to fishing with the *giop* sailing ships which, like their crews, also partly originate from outside – from the North Moluccan maritime sphere.[6]

Starting with the early activities of the Dutch Missionary Society (NZG) in the 1840s, Amurang like the rest of the Minahasan peninsula was extensively Christianized and westernized.[7] Like other colonizers, the Dutch complained about the general state of hygiene and health, housing conditions and heavy workloads of pregnant women. Due to measures like introducing vaccinations, both the general state of health and population numbers rose steadily, while infant mortality dropped (Schouten 1993:65–9). According to the 1930 Census, in Amurang there were 47 'children not yet able to walk' per hundred adult women, at which time Amurang had a considerably higher fertility and/or lower infant mortality than Java and Sumatra (Jones 1977:105–6).

In 1919 the Borgo were naturalized with the indigenes (Watuseke 1968:57). Today they are still proud of their mestizo backgrounds, believing that they are partly of European descent. Borgo identity is based on links with outsiders. They think they are the closest a Minahasan can become to the 'clever', 'modern' and 'advanced' Europeans: in their outlook and as original converts to Christianity. Colonial history prepared Minahasans for a flexible attitude towards cultural imports, ever since derogatorily defined as 'mimicking the West' (Hickson 1889; Bucholt 1994). Yet both Christianity and institutional education are central to what it is to be a Minahasan and to live with 'a tradition of change' (Lundström-Burghoorn 1981). These factors are necessary to appreciate the fairly close match between Amurang *giop* fishermen's ethnomedical conceptions of physical substances transmitted at conception and the modern, national knowledge available locally through health centres, the mass media and education.

THE CHILD'S ENTRY INTO THE WORLD

In the village of Bitung, fishermen's houses cluster in rows parallel to the beach, along the narrow coastline. These rows reflect the economic differentials between the houses, each of which forms an economically independent household built around a core cohabiting couple: the row nearest the sea consists of the poorest fishing huts of canoe fishers and young families of *giop* crewmembers. These suffer from occasional destruction by high waves. *Tanta*[8] Agu, who is a Sangir-born widowed 68-year-old mother of three, lives there. She is a traditional midwife (*dukun*) in third generation and, like the rest of the neighbourhood, a Protestant Christian. The subsequent row of houses contains wealthier, established households with *giop* captains, owners and non-fishers. *Tanta* Ina, a 78-year-old *mama biang*, lives there. She bore five children besides the two who died in infancy. At the time when her Borgo husband was not yet a village head and she was nearing forty, women 'called and called for her', because 'they saw I was brave'. Like *Tanta* Agu, she also works outside her immediate area of residence, from the present Borgo stronghold Bitung to the former Borgo quarters now known as the villages of Uwuran I and Ranoyapo. Now, her disciples are her eldest daughter and her daughter-in-law, who stand in for her when her health fails.

Tanta Agu and *Tanta* Ina start cooperating with a pregnant woman in a leisurely manner immediately after their help is sought. In such 'brave' (*brani*) hands, a woman who seeks to conceive or to get help during her pregnancy and labour is safe. A woman who fails to get pregnant is told to eat rich foods such as honey and stop working or worrying too much. She has to seek 'strength (*kekuatan*) of the body'. 'Medicinal waters', which consist of boiled water mixed with leaves and roots of various kinds, are essential. After establishing that the time of her period has just passed, a midwife comes to massage her and continues to do so periodically. Massages enhance fertility and concentrate on her breasts and especially the stomach which may have 'fallen down' or be 'too weak'. Midwives claim they can tell this from the outward shape. To prepare herself for pregancy or to aid a period of gestation already begun, a woman takes egg-yolks[9] of chicken mixed with finely pounded turmeric (*kuning*) or drinks *saguer*, the sweet and mildly alcoholic sap of the sugar palm (*seho*). A husband should satisfy his pregnant wife's dietary wishes ('he'd better provide, for God help the marriage if he doesn't'). Her food cravings are compared to the insatiable hunger for fish of the best *giop* vessels.[10]

Babies are thought to become boys or girls by chance, 'just in their own right'. Parents simply wish that their baby will be 'strong'. The sex of the baby is an object of speculation, although of little anxiety. Borgo parents acknowledge that by a curious chance of biology, sometimes babies are born who have blue eyes, rather fair reddish hair, or a sharp and high 'European' nose, even a skin a degree 'whiter'. These are considered beautiful and received as delightful evidence that there is 'European descent' (*turunan Eropa*) in the family. A Ranoyapo boy was born with six toes on each foot. A man from the same village has six fingers on one hand. These are coveted Borgo anomalies, even signs of special qualities.

The number of temporary occupants in a house where there is illness or a pregant woman increases considerably. Before birth, close kinswomen and neighbours share work. After the birth, the cost of treating guests is covered on a voluntary basis by these same people (cf. Lundström 1976). Most pregnant women prefer to move to their mother's house for giving birth. Those who are pregnant for the first time are usually still living either with their own mother or in the house of their mother-in-law. Birth preparations are not singled out as the female domain only. Nor are men's roles in them elaborated. A *giop* captain with a pregnant wife organized the labour-intensive maintenance work of his boat to coincide with the estimated time of birth, so as not to be at sea. Ideally husbands stay around until the umbilical cord drops and refrain from fishing for seven days. In practice, economic pressures override this rule.

When the time of labour comes, the midwife takes over and gives instructions to the few kinswomen present. The nervous husband stays around in the compound, or helps his wife by holding her from underneath her armpits. *Tanta* Ina gives coffee to the woman in labour, 'because it makes the child come out more quickly'. Each of the traditional midwives 'uses' her own esoteric knowledge (*ilmu*), and they can be understood tacitly to compete with each other. *Tanta* Agu gives medicinal water (*obat air*) which 'is not from human sources', with the implication that it is from the ancestors, the 'very old people of yesterday'. All healers and midwives blow (*tiop*) this ancestral help onto the patient, 'where it hurts'. *Tanta* Ina scoffs at this and simply gives her water in a drinking glass. She stresses her practical experience and reliance on God to whom she prays, and suggests her customers give alms in church. Women who are 'in torture' will 'ask and ask' for medicinal waters, which they are given. In fact, much of midwives' discourse lingers around the theme of women 'pleading for' (*minta*) their help, which they give at any time, by any means, forgetting themselves.

After the birth, the mother is massaged and bathed daily by the midwife, and so is the infant, who receives the 'little bath' with a cloth dipped into warm water. Special leaves are used in the bathwater, such as the small bitter lemon (*lemong suangi*) which also, when attached to the swaddled infant, wards off nocturnal evils. Another bathwater ingredient is *dandang* leaf which is said to have 'electricity', which implies physical strength. 'To make her happy and her body lightweight (*ringan*) and strong (*kuat*)', the mother is given finely pounded *goraka* root to drink. Many women said that it is important that female friends keep the new mother company. She might have all kinds of problems which will not be helped by having to 'stay inside all alone'. In previous years, the new mother would remain indoors for forty days, seeing only people who came to visit her, before going to church. It is said today that if she goes to church before this time has lapsed, she may not take Holy Communion.

Both mother and baby are stroked gently with hands warmed by a slowly burning hearth (*raho diapi*, *bara*), which was built before the labour in the room reserved for it. The mother and the baby sleep by the fire. The house must be protected because 'bad winds' (*angin jahat*) can smell the blood of childbirth. Strenuous labour causes loss of blood which results in a 'sense of cold' (*rasa dingin*) and make the body weak (*lemah*). (Men at sea also see their tiring fishing and lack of drinking water as resulting in loss of blood (*darah*)). Blood is a measure of strength. Mothers worry about keeping themselves and the child so 'warm' that they 'sweat and (one's) face becomes red'. This kind of controlled heating is different from the unhealthy heat of fever and infections. 'Heating' or 'warming up' (*kase panas*) prevents the infant's stomach from becoming tough and stiff, or 'hot' (*panas*), which is more or less the same as *rigor mortis*. Excessive heat only results in death. After several days, the mother might be seen sitting by her front door with the baby on her lap, while she transfers the heat of her palms warmed above a bowl of hot coals to the baby's body. This goes on until the stump of the umbilical cord drops. Uncontrolled cooling is a sign of diminished alertness and invites attacks across the unguarded ever-permeable boundaries – of babies, adults, boats and houses.

A baby is swathed from armpits to hips in a white rectangular cloth (*gurita*), which protects it. Except when washing the baby, the mother will keep it tied thus with many strings over the torso for about three months. One new mother said that the *gurita* 'prevents a baby from eating too much as some are born big because the mother drank too much palm sap'. An ex-guerilla of the Permesta insurgency told me that during the early 1960s he wore a *gurita* hidden underneath his shirt. Another man, a soldier enrolled in the Indonesian army, uses a *gurita* in East Timor, because he is afraid for his life. If for them the removal of the *gurita* marked an ending of a dangerous period, perhaps for a neonate it signs the beginning of its chance of survival?

SOULS AND HEALTH

Post-natal care of infants and mothers is largely concerned with protection. This is about re-establishing balance by removing all traces of upset and blood. The anxiety about washing the bloody clothes (by the husband or a kinswoman) and about cleaning the bloody placenta and umbilical cord 'until they almost shine' is not a result of a concern for purity and pollution. Blood literally 'smells' (*bau-bau*) of weakness and illness.[11] Blood may attract Pontianak, a bad spirit with human origin (*roh jahat*) who is more feared than ghosts (*hantu*) or the devil (*iblis, satan*). Pontianak is a woman who bled to death in childbirth. Thirsty for blood, she may lure unsuspecting men with her beauty and attack them. A captain's wife told me how in her birth village Motoling she once attended the funeral of a woman who bled to death after labour. The corpse's hair was nailed between the coffin lid and container so that she would not return to bother the living.

Since then, she hovers above the ground with her intestines protruding out of a headless neck.

Babies (*bayi*) enter the world still weak and vulnerable to the vagaries of black magic by malevolent people, the devil, bad spirits and infant diseases. The infant's fontanel is covered with 'protecting leaves' against the soul-loss which could result from being startled. Mothers are susceptible to 'dizziness' (*pusing*). Some use a white cloth tied around their forehead. Nothing much is fixed about the babies as yet, not even the certainty of their survival. Apart from their gender, not even the social status of infants is fixed by birth, as fishermen tend to deny intrinsic differences among people. In customs related to infant rearing, boys and girls are treated similarly, the chief exception being that parents buy blue clothes for boys and pink ones for girls. Later on, children will gradually learn the signs and practical pathways towards *sumangat*, an embodied vitality both physical and spiritual which is necessary for success in any undertaking. People who behave 'with *sumangat*' are 'potent' (they accomplish) because they are 'spirited' (alert).[12]

The infant, whose life force is 'not yet stable', will need his/her spiritual 'younger sibling' (*ade*) which is the placenta. This 'younger sibling' shares in the infant's soul-substance and is his/her 'friend'. The two are born within minutes or hours of each other: this almost abolishes the difference of birth order, which creates status differences between siblings. Graafland ([1869]1991:115–16) tells how in old Minahasa every child was thought to have a 'protective spirit' against sickness and evil, who was 'born together' with the child. Its name was 'of same age' (*rengarengan*).

The neonate and its placenta are the two inseparable sides of new life which has become embodied, when the parents gave them their material substance (*badan*, body). This is not gendered, or derived from either mother or the father, or from female or male forefathers.[13] At the moment of the birth, God gave the baby a soul (*roh*) from heaven. Yet another component could be thought of as 'life force' because this is found in all living animals, plants and humans: the child and its placenta, besides having shared in the same matter before the birth, continue to share their 'spirit' or 'animating force' (*jiwa*). Perhaps it is the *jiwa* which in its active and autonomous aspect could be called the 'breath of life'. This is because people talk about the invisible world, coterminous with the earth and God's heaven, as the 'air' (*langi-langi*) which is infested with 'winds' (*angin*) and 'clouds' (*awan*). Sent by malevolent people, these try to 'enter' and substitute for, or diminish, the soul-substance (*jiwa*) of an infant or a patient. Thus a person exists where the soul-substances and a body temporarily coincide but the components may be added to or lost. Death comes when *jiwa* departs from a body. Also this is a process which takes some time, and it is finalized by the mourners' ceremonies of 'remembrance'. After the physical death *roh* simply 'goes back to God'.

THE BURIAL OF THE 'SIBLING' AND COMPENSATING FOR MIDWIFE'S CARE

Like the infant, the placenta is washed and packed up into a tight 'parcel' by the midwife. The inner brown hard husk of a coconut is chopped into fine shreds which are applied as a medicine for the stump of the umbilical cord. Parents will also have chosen the inner husk of another coconut, with two 'beautiful' halves. This becomes the container in which the midwife places the washed placenta with 'medicines'. She then leaves the house and, accompanied by the father, chooses a corner of the yard of the house where she buries the placenta while uttering a spell or Christian prayer. They must walk there straightaway, 'without glancing to left or right, otherwise the baby will grow up a timid adult with eyes pointing here and there'. Each person's afterbirth, which is buried in the yard, will 'always draw one back' and remind one how the parents cared for him/her. Some of my informants belittled their act as 'just a habit'.

Both midwives charge for these services. They are compensated seven days after labour, or when the infant's umbilical cord drops away. This marks the moment when the midwife's responsibility for the infant ceases. When her follow-up services are not needed anymore, she literally takes her hands off (*lepas tangan*) the baby. She receives a meal as lavish as possible and her fee, which is sometimes no more than a plastic bag of rice, vegetables and sweet potatoes to take home for cooking. The remunerations involved are not discussed openly. Instead, women know fairly well what *Tanta* Agu or *Tanta* Ina will charge. The former will be pleased to be fed cookies and tea (customary treatment for guests of honour) and expects to be paid according to the mother's means, between Rp. 7,000 and 20,000. *Tanta* Ina is more expensive, but she too will accept fish, cloth or other 'gifts' in kind, or from around Rp. 35,000 upwards.[14] Many women are afraid of *Tanta* Agu, because she is also commissioned for love magic. It was rumoured that she had resorted to hurting a baby by black magic when shamed by lack of respect or the undue modesty of a payment. Supposedly, she had kept on 'holding' (*pegang*) the infant, who then died. The stress placed on the treatment of the placenta and the importance of paying for, or 'balancing' (*balas*), the midwife's care open up issues about the sources of human well-being.

'MEDICINES OF THE LAND'

Nonetheless, the infant has internal 'strength' of its own, shared with the 'younger sibling'. That is why the umbilical cord (*tali pusat*) has invigorating powers. It was the life-line between the infant and its placenta. Therefore it is dried and made into a medicine (*obat tali pusat*) by storing it in a powder box. On demand, fine shavings of it are mixed with boiled water. Inserting the stump into powder gives the powder healing qualities for treating the infant's navel against inflammations.[15]

The medical efficacy of roots, leaves, fruits and nuts is based on their origins in the land, which is itself fertile. The 'medicines of the land' (*obat makatanah*) are the living ingredients of the land whose fertility provides an assurance of continuity. People trust the good-will of ancestors, who 'are still all around, they know, they see' because 'we haven't lost contact with them' and 'we still listen to their teachings'. Perhaps even the umbilical cord medicine has an ancestor-related rationale as a repository of life force. I was not treated with 'medicines of the land' until after a long stay in Amurang, 'because there is no way of telling that they are not poison' to a foreigner. A considerable time had to elapse before people decided that I qualified for 'Minahasan medicines', that they would 'agree' with me.

Healers and midwives not only appeal to the intrinsic potencies of the plants, but are also experienced in what we call the chemically effective ingredients: papaya leaves and seeds protect from malaria, the roots and branches of both the wild 'forest tomato' and *kumis kucing* help in kidney dysfunctions (TAD 1987). Schefold (1995) has studied the efficacy of plants in healing and protecting in Indonesia. In Amurang, too, plants have intrinsic powers by virtue of their names, their morphological characteristics, growing places or outward resemblances in form, shape or colour to either human ailments or to the desired results. For example, a leaf whose name evokes sturdiness is applied in oil and massaged on the skin for healing fractured bones. The most potent healing ingredients are rare and originate from far-away places where fishermen have travelled, even from peoples of other religious denominations on the coasts of Central Sulawesi.[16] People's faith in them is not unquestioned, but 'it would be silly not to try every possible means' – healers, 'shop medicines' and prayers. I was told that the effects of the 'medicines of the land' last longer: one drinks three glasses of 'water' on three consecutive days, instead of doctor's pills (*obat dokter*) which are taken every few hours. Besides, modern medicines are only obtained at cost from the pharmacy, whereas traditional medicines share many characteristics which make them readily available and practical to use. Houses have vegetable plots with plants which have healing properties, a 'living pharmacy' (*apotik hidop*). Some of them grow wild and one simply has to know where to search.

MARRIAGE AS MUTUAL CARE

A carer's labour of nursing and healing places debts upon the child or on any other person receiving it. Protection, care and maintenance (*piara*) and their mutuality are salient idioms in relation to both marriage and childcare. Before looking at the multiple kinds of childcare arrangements, we need to understand the nature of Amurang marriage. It is because of children that people – sometimes – have their marriage legalized. The shared responsibility over children makes a union permanent.[17] People only become adults, that is 'responsible', through parenthood. Childless adults cannot yet be addressed with adult terms of reference and they should partake in those local savings and credit associations and Christian meetings designated for adolescents. Children are the meaning of life and insurance for old age.

A majority of the cohabiting Bitung fishermen answered affirmatively to my question 'are you already married (so*kawin*)?' For a time, I was puzzled over the level of wedding ceremonies completed, until a pun by a fisherman taught me that my 'findings' were useless. According to him he had 'married often, but never married'.[18] He played with the nuances of the two words for 'marriage': one (*kawin*) could mean 'to sleep together' unless more specified, and the other (*nikah*) means a legal marriage, filed at the civil registry office and blessed by the church (*kawin gereja*). The latter is the only legally binding marriage (*kawin sah*). So all along, these couples had confirmed that they had children, instead of embarrassing me by rephrasing the question into 'do you already have a family (*soberkeluarga*)?' which was what they expected to be asked. Furthermore, they were reluctant either to disclose their lack of funds for an official marriage ceremony or to use the local phrase for cohabitation. Christian fishermen typically live in arrangements which they laughingly call 'mutual care' or 'keeping each other'[19] (*bakupiara*). This reciprocal verb is also used of domestic animals such as pigs and dogs. Like animals, people take care of their offspring without legal arrangements.

Fishermen relish jokes, word-plays and sexual innuendos. Sex is talked about as 'playing' (*main-main*). Although positively valued, affectionate behaviour is muted in public. For both sexes, walking outside *alone* after dark suggests clandestine affairs. 'Running here and there' (*lari kesana kamari*) is frowned upon. It happens though, because normally the 'marriage', which people say should be a private affair between the two young people, is settled when the girl becomes pregnant. This consummation of a relationship ideally suggests a creation of a morally binding union based on 'mutual love/pity' (*bakusayang*) between and across the generations. If faced with parental opposition, the lovers will even try the symbolic 'marriage by running' (*kawin lari*).[20] People then say that 'it's already happened' (*sojadi*), meaning that the youngsters could have had time for intercourse. The couple then establishes an economically independent household of their own, within the house of either of their parents, before they have funds to build their own house.

Although Minahasans reckon kinship in a cognatic fashion, surnames are inherited patrilineally. Thus children born outside legal marriage receive their mother's surname. This causes some older couples to suddenly take part in the periodically church-organized 'mass marriages' (*kawin masal*) for poor people. An elder Borgo couple who got married in their late fifties explained that this ensured that their son (who was himself about to marry) would pass on his father's Borgo surname to the eventual children. Had the old couple a daughter intending to marry, she would pass her father's surname to the name tag above the main entrance of her future house. For Borgo families this is important, although they no longer have special endogamous marriage preferences, as remembered by the oldest generation. The practical acceptance of paternity overrides the need to bless the spouses' union in church, which in any case is prohibitively expensive for most fishermen. Babies are considered as much the infants of their absent fathers as they are of their mothers. But the judgement regarding women who are single parents is: 'her own fault'; 'No marriage, no money (from the man)'.

Fishermen see the conjugal couple as equal partners in the new household, and their children, regardless of sex, as equal receivers of what little there is to inherit. Further symmetry in both legalized and common-law marriages is suggested, because in divorce neither spouse is entitled to the children automatically. Only if they are very small does their mother keep them. In the past, according to Minahasan *adat* law, parents' equal rights over keeping the children and rights to their labour were overshadowed, or complemented, by a notion that children belonged to the mother's kin-group until her bridewealth had been paid in full. Again, as with midwives, this is an example of care reciprocated in money. During the course of the nineteenth century the missionaries managed to change what they saw as 'brideprice' into a bride's personal gift, by refusing to bless marriages which involved 'brideprice'. Until then, the bridewealth would, among other things, 'open up children's eyes' so that they recognized their father, acting as a compensation for the bride's family for her lost reproductive and productive capacities. It gave the children the right to inherit from their father. Its full payment symbolized the unification of the spouses into a 'connecting stem' from which new generations could sprout (van Bemmelen 1992:182–4).[21]

CARE AS A MEDIUM OF KINSHIP

Care underlines the issue of whom the child belongs to and therefore it has cultural and economic consequences. When pressed by me, *Ibu*[22] Sartje, a captain's wife, reluctantly separated her adopted son from her biological children, by saying that he was not 'child of one womb' (*anak sekandung*), then more radically, not 'true/actual child' (*anak sunggu*). The point is that she disliked being pressed so far. The biological parents of this boy were her husband's crewmember and his wife, who had judged that they could not afford this seventh child.

Sometimes also one's siblings' adopted or fostered children are called 'true children'. Most of them are 'still one "family" [*keluarga*], one blood [*darah*]' with their adoptive parents because they are the bilateral cousins of their new step-siblings. The word 'still' is important here. Unity gets mixed with the diversity of new connections, new blood. Slowly, each successive generation shares less and less matter with their cognatic forebears. This historic aspect of kinship is manifested in the many overlapping, non-corporate descent groups (*turunan*). Equally, the dilution of relatedness happens horizontally with contemporary kin: everyone belongs to several cognatic, non-corporate kin-groups (*keluarga*) of his/her living relatives with whom affinity or biological relatedness is shared. The sameness of 'blood' is a vague open-ended continuum used to downplay or underline differences with those who are remote (*jauh*) or close (*dekat*). In this sense 'blood' comes to signify not blood as such, but 'the possibility to contrast the sharers of a common heredity with others who lack the ability to trace relationship in that sense' (Lundström-Burghoorn 1981:129–31).

Breast milk is another medium which creates enduring bonds. It is a prototypical means of care. Milk defines all parties involved as kin and those at the receiving end as siblings. Marriage between bilateral first cousins is abhored. People objected by saying 'They are almost like siblings!'. This implies that in theory they could have suckled at the same breast. It makes their intermarriage as close relatives unthinkable. When contrasted with other people who belong to either the same classificatory or real generation (*tingkat*), this dense cluster is called 'the generation of milk siblings (*susunan*). Marriage between second cousins is neither ruled out nor desirable. Instead of actual age, it is the commonality of real or potential receipt of care (like milk) which defines each generational level. It separates groups of people into feeders and those fed. The ties of milk which united children were also important in the past An old indigenous word *sanatotoan*[23] meant 'family'. It 'derived from *toto*, "milk" ... signifying "they who have drunk, sucked, of the same milk"' (Wilken 1921:58; also Hickson 1889:284).

Ibu Sartje had only one child (a daughter) to whom she had given birth herself. She then had a miscarriage quite late into her second pregnancy. Later she gave birth to twins who both died within days. She then adopted the baby boy mentioned on p. 102. For her and other women, long-term (breast)feeding is an idiom for self-sacrifice and disinterested care. Women say babies suck away their 'strength'. *Ibu* Sartje declared: 'But I gave him everything I had, all my money went to buying the tinned milk (*susu bleik*). I didn't bother about the powder milk, just tinned. Isn't he now as if my own son?' In addition to tinned milk given to her boy, I think she was stressing the efforts and the money she had invested in him.

AMURANG ADOPTION AND FOSTERAGE

As an extension of relatedness created through care, adoptions of many kinds may substitute for birth. An explanation for the frequent divorces is 'mutual incompatibility' (*nganda bakucocok*). My material does not confirm the decisive role of childlessness, reported elsewhere in Indonesia, but broken relationships are issues which people are quiet about. An unusual example would be a couple who waited for ten years before the woman conceived. People resort to adoptions to counteract infertility just as they adopt children because of responsibilities towards kin. A woman's acceptance of an adoption is necessary and supports my view that women have a firm standing *vis-à-vis* their husbands.[24] The few official and many unofficial caring arrangements fit well with the reality of extra-marital children.[25] Responsibility for the welfare of children lies also with grandparents, nearby relatives and long-term fishing companions. They feel obliged to keep an eye on them and offer them food or a place to stay overnight if the child so wants. Here also the generational, cognatic nature of Amurang kinship becomes visible. The role of horizontal kin (siblings and first cousins) is primary. Typically, siblings or grandparents of either spouse ask for a toddler whose 'face' they like. From the child's point of view, the transaction is smoothly concluded. Young boys even suggest it themselves, if they get into arguments with their parents.

In Amurang there are many names for fosterage and adoptions, which roughly equal the practical differences in arrangements. The village government is notified of a legalized adoption certified by a court. Adopted children (*anak adopsi/angkat*) should become full members of their new household and receive the same rights of inheritance as the biological children.

A sickly child receives a new nickname or parents start using his/her baptismal name. Names are important and they have to 'match mutually' (*bakucocok*) with the person carrying them. If a child fails to thrive, parents give him/her away for a while to one of their siblings, for fosterage. A child 'lifted up' (*anak angkat*) is a fostered child, whose biological parents gave him/her to another house because of health problems during early childhood. A reason for a child to be 'thrown away' (*anak buang*) is again similar, that is, frequent illness in the house of the biological parents.

The most typical rendering for long-term fosterage is *anak piara*, a 'cared-for child'. S/he is a 'child raised like one's own'.[26] *Piara* means to 'protect, raise or rear'. If a couple has more children than they can afford, they may give one away. Some poorer families would hand a pre-adolescent boy or girl to their better-off friends in the neighbourhood, in return for shelter and food. Such a boy would fish with his new temporary family, while a girl would do household work and be pleased to get some nice clothing. This arrangement augments friendships and helps to widen important networks, originally created at sea between a captain and his crew, or on land between boat owners, fish dealers and captains.

The love and care given to an *anak piara* make him/her like *anak mengaku*, a child who is confessed to or 'claimed to be one's own'. To support the status of such an admitted child, there might be a private 'letter' signed by both parties. *Ibu* Sartje objected bitterly when her son's biological mother started to visit her house. Five years earlier, when her husband carried the barely 14-day-old infant to their house, an ultimate security was a 'letter', filed away in their house. It stated the amount of compensation the biological parents had received and was signed by both parties. Few differences appear between *anak piara* and *anak mengaku*, whose adoptive parents become his/her legal parents. Otherwise they appear to be interchangeable terms. Like any children who do not go to school, both work fully for their households. Interestingly, in the past *anak mengaku* was a child whose natural parents remained her/his legal parents. Adoption was a 'business-like relationship' because the adopters needed labour. Later on, this became 'a contract of care' whereby, against the child's future labour input, s/he would inherit from both sets of parents (Gandhi-Lapian 1995:101).

In ancient Minahasa to 'acknowledge a child', known in Amurang as *piki anak*, was a public affair concluded by a joint feast between the two parties. Adoption did not only concern children. Parents sought to adopt other adults of higher status. The adopters were of lower status and promised to work for the adoptee. The adoptee, in return, promised political support and would in time inherit from his adopters (Graafland [1869]1991:271; Carpentier Alting 1901:133–43; Lundström-Burghoorn 1981:63). In today's Amurang the preference for multiple Christian godparents for one's child needs to be seen in this light. Schouten (1993:86) notes that what Europeans in Minahasa took to be adoptions were about protection, access to labour and land – in short, creation of dyadic patron–client relationships. Among the Christian Toraja of Central Sulawesi they have politico-economic consequences: adoptions may give rise to debt relations, which are counted in buffaloes (Volkman 1985:95; cf. Schrauwers 1995:350). Among Malaysian fishermen children's adoptive and caring arrangements are an important aspect in the local creation of community (Carsten 1991). Amurang missionaries fostered or adopted some of their young local disciples (Graafland [1869]1991:297; Schouten 1993:117, 1995), an arrangement for religious education which the ancient Minahasan female or male priests (*walian*) used for passing on their knowledge and powers (Bucholt 1994:19). This is a system of knowledge transfer familiar to today's midwives, whose disciples preferably are younger relatives. The relationship is a hierarchical one and based on differences of age and generation. It is defined as a parent–child relationship which is a model for mutually beneficial arrangements between parties who are in many ways unequal.

CONCLUSION

The interrelated themes evoked underpin the different meanings that Amurang childbirth gains in a plurality of contexts. Depending on the midwife's personal approach, the 'religion of yesterday' is more or less influenced by local Protestant Christianity. Western knowledge, admired by the Borgo, gives credit to midwives like *Tanta* Ina, with her certificate from a formal course she has undertaken. There is clearly a dual system of healing in operation, due to the exclusion of local concepts from the formal health-care sector and the expense of the latter. In cases of arrested labour, *Tanta* Ina sends the woman to the local hospital, but a cost of one hospital bed per night may be as high as a fisherman's monthly income. There is no 'heating' either in hospitals. Hospitalized mothers worry about how to get the placenta home.

Secondly, Amurang understandings of the origins of life and the many 'soul-substances' which come together to form a new human being are in several ways typically Southeast Asian. There is nothing singularly Minahasan about the practice of 'heating' mothers, about the belief in Pontianak and other concerns for blood, or about the technical processes of childbirth and burial of the placenta (Laderman 1987; Errington 1989:38–40; Carsten 1992, 1995). Health and disease are conceptualized as depending on the state of souls (Errington 1983; Laderman 1991). Also Amurang birth practices concentrate on the presence of soul-substances and how steadily anchored they are within the body. Illnesses and ailments identified are ultimately attributed to this. 'Strength' and stamina cannot be achieved unless also 'the mind is happy'. Bowen has treated the visible and invisible processes of birth beautifully, as 'pathways' into 'embodiment' and 'empowerment' among the Muslim Gayo highlanders of north Sumatra, and his material bears a resemblance to Minahasa (1993:118–22, 218–23). In Amurang, the *jiwa*, which is divided between the infant and the placenta, shows that a person consists not only of the body, which will learn to display the signs of integration and intensiveness (*sumangat*),[27] but also of a non-predetermined quantity of invisible soul-substances. Of special relevance here is Karsten's definition of *jiwa* as a sensitive soul-stuff which 'ebbs away with the blood' and which is 'ascribed to the placenta' (1935:49–50).[28]

A third issue is the place of metaphorical language and its selectiveness in a given culture. To what extent, asks Dube in her study of the 'seed' and 'earth' metaphors in northern and central India, 'can the cultural conception of human reproductive process expressed in the metaphorical language ... be viewed as a part of ethno-science?' (1986:34). Such is the problem of the 'personal agents' or the 'winds' sent by malevolent or envious Amurang people. It is also a problem with the extreme and therefore dangerous 'hotness' (*panas*) vs. extreme 'coldness' (*dingin*), and with the moderate and therefore healthy 'warmth' (*panas)* vs. moderate 'coolness' (*dingin*). The transparent meanings of bodily temperatures and of 'heating' are evident. Potentially they are humoral idioms referring to the states of the vital substances like blood (whether diminished or not in the material or spiritual universe), as much as they are shorthand for a midwife's project of fixing the mental and physical equilibrium, and ways of referring to people who deal with it (as when Amurang midwives are said to have 'cool hands').

Moreover, midwives also manage social and psychological problems and find rationalizations for the disparities between body and mind. These present themselves as loss of 'equilibrium', as a sort of disorientation a 'dizzy' mother is experiencing. Wikan (1990) writes about the vagaries of being upset and how people struggle to learn the right emotions. The (a) imbalance results in (b) the visible disease or a threat of it, and is therefore as important to identify and heal by a midwife's folk-psychiatry, as is the body which is treated with 'doctor's medicines' and 'brave' hands. Symptomatically, early anthropology took this to be 'magico-religious', failing to understand that, excluding bricoleurs and imposters, the best healers are far from being 'non-secular'. They are just as likely to chant or give amulets and to incorporate a whole family into the healing seance, as they are to prescribe and apply medicines, massages, etc., based on long experience. They understand the uncertainty of maternal well-being and infant survival. Indeed, the Indonesian maternal and infant mortality rates are high.[29] Among the Wana of eastern central Sulawesi the semantic differentiation between different words for 'baby' marks the stages of a neonate's viability and the chances of its survival (Atkinson 1996:173). The timing and usage of the *gurita* cloth in Amurang appear to follow this logic. Recently in *Anthropology Today*, Wall has criticized the tendency to badly over-culturalize what are the non-mythical and folk bio-medical childbirth issues. The eagerness to disregard the 'rational' complex in favour of the 'magical' one might lead to unnecessary reification of our own anecdotal experience, and into equally misplaced glorification of such instances when we study foreign cultures (1995:12–17).

One local way to present the dilemma is the debt for care and life, the obligatory reciprocity which defines the relationship of a new mother to her midwife. The mother is obliged to 'balance', otherwise the relationship between the transactors is severed and a possibility of retribution arises. This felt ambiguity defines particularly the relationship a mother has to a traditional midwife who is a 'life deliverer' by virtue of her secret ancestral knowledge. Here reproduction and the non-definitive character of maternal or infant's blood as it partly signifies spiritual well-being are dependent on a midwife's benevolent care. Respect and thankfulness directed towards ancestors for their medicines and to people with healing skills are important. Spouses come to be 'married' when they decide to 'mutually take care of each other' as they have a baby to care for. Moral behaviour is formulated around mutual help which results in the indebtedness of children. Adoption and fosterage are based on the idiom of care and nurturance, such as mother's milk or tinned milk given by a woman to a child she considers her own. On top of the notions of shared relatedness through substances like blood and breast milk, which Carsten (1995) shows to be interrelated, I have sought to show how care itself contributes towards relatedness. People come to be defined as the generation who provided care, or as the generation on the receiving end. Within each generation, a core unit of relatives seems to be a group of siblings and bilateral first cousins, who potentially have been breastfeed by the same woman, who cannot intermarry and who foster each other's children. It remains to be seen how these debts, in their widest economic, social and political sense, bind Amurang fishermen together.

Finally, the disparities between what Amurang people say they do, and what they actually do, are not always due to 'political correctness'. Instead, the cultural explanations and the actual health care in the western bio-medical sense are two incommensurable ways of dealing with an important event, the birth of a child. They do not come into conflict with each other. Although interlinked, even causally connected, they ultimately address the problem of birth with separate modes of rationalization: one with the logic of practice, the other with the logic of explaining further by applying meaning to practice. The physical fact that each human being is born with its placenta is meaningfully rephrased as the birth of siblings – thus expressing the primacy of siblingship and its sustenance. This goes on long after the two 'friends' are separated by birth and long before this process is deemed successful.

NOTES

1 Fieldwork in 1995–6 was sponsored by the Indonesian Institute of Science (LIPI), Jakarta, and the Faculty of Letters, Sam Ratulangi University, Manado. Project funding comes from the Academy of Finland, Council for Culture and Society, and the Nordic Institute of Asian Studies (NIAS), Copenhagen. Thanks for comments are due to Kari Grøtterud, Peter van Eeuwijk and the participants of the LSE Anthropology Department Writing-Up Seminar, especially to Amina Abu Shebab. In Manado, I wish to thank Tante Lus Ranty-Politton, Drs Alex Ulaen and Drs Frans S. Watuseke with their families. In Amurang, I owe every fish caught and sold to the *giop* captain Tona'as Nyong 'Tou', his family and neighbours.

2 *Puskesmas*: *Pusat Kesejahteraan Keluarga* (lit. Family Health Centre).

3 As in Amurang, in Java, a *dukun* is a healer/herbalist, skilled in massage and exorcizing bad spirits (Boomgaard 1993:86, 1996:50, 76). In Indonesia varied types of *dukun*, or traditional healers, are known, although their functions and skills vary (Slamet-Velsink 1996:76).

4 'Traditional' means fishing which is mostly small-scale, family-based and beach-landing, as opposed to the salaried off-shore fishers with trawlers in the city of Bitung on the Minahasan south coast. Raymond Firth [1946]1966) has argued for the rationality of subsistence fishers which places them within the category of 'peasants'.

5 In Amurang there are a few Muslim and some Catholic Borgo people. An oral history of one Borgo kin-group traces its background to a high-ranking Tidorean lady.

6 In Ternate, Tidore and Ambon where there also were Christian 'freed people', *giop* vessels are known as *rorehe*, or (in Dutch documents) as *orembaai*. Amurang captains know that the *rorehe* vessel got its local name 'giop' from its larger purse-seine (the *giop* net) for catching small tuna. Dutch measures for maritime pacification, the *rorehe* and the Borgo are linked in a manuscript by a former Resident of Manado, A.J. van Olpen (1843, 1844–6).

7 According to J. Kroeskamp (1974), Minahasa had the highest literacy rate and density of schools in the Netherlands Indies, even when compared with the important Java. For an excellent study on how 'Minahasa' was created, see Henley (1992).

8 *Tanta*, 'aunt', 'auntie'. The honorific, but slightly informal title of Dutch origin for women elder then ego, who usually belong to the eldest, grandparental generation.

9 For countering love magic (*ilmu sayang*), that is, anti-love magic, rotten eggs are used.

10 In this paper I do not have space to spell out all the parallels between land and sea activities. It is widely accepted that *giop* vessels are captains' 'second women'. The 'medicinal waters' also feature in *giop* healing. Some are fortified with esoteric spells or with woodfilings of a captain's medicinal woods. Also eggs, turmeric and palm vine (distilled into the strong spirit *cap tikus*) are used. The purpose of 'fixing

a boat' is ideally to make its belly, the midships, as full as a pregnant woman's.

11 Graafland ([1869]1991:95, 103) describes one of the now extinct traditional Minahasan sacrifical feasts (*foso*). This *foso* was held for a person who was under pressure because of sickness. In this ritual the sick person drank animal blood, which was associated with calming down and getting rid of disease.

12 The Tontemboan word *kĕtĕr* refers to a 'religiously charged' notion of 'inner force' (Schouten 1993:24–8). '*Kĕtĕr*' is virtually unknown in Amurang where coastal Malay has replaced Tontemboan. One major difference apart (that fact that in the highlands *kĕtĕr* could be inherited), the word 'potency' perhaps underlines the convergences between *sumangat* and *kĕtĕr*. A classic study of *sumange* is Anderson (1972).

13 Cf. the notions of soft female and hard male substances in Madagaskar, in Bloch (1992) and Carsten (1995) and Thomas (this volume).

14 In 1995 this was the equivalent of one-third of an average fisherman's monthly income or three-quarters of the price of a monthly bag of rice enough for a family of four.

15 The navel of the *giop*, a hole made at the joint of the keel, is where the ship's animation springs from. When a Christian boat owner uses a Muslim or traditionalist shipwright, a little piece of wood will be cut from the ship and buried in a secret place, so that the boat will 'find its way back home'. On the Muslim inter-island traders in southeast Sulawesi, see Southon (1995).

16 People also seek help from the giop captains (*tona'as*), who from their fishing trips are known to stock charms and medicines: wood, roots, black coral and ambergris.

17 Children fix their parents' position as a possible new focal point of a *turunan* (cognatic non-corporate descent group) of future generations. In old Minahasa a man had no membership in his wife's family until he had produced children. The spouses became kin only when they had children (Hickson 1889:281; cf. Carsten 1992). Also among the Kaili-Pamona of Central Sulawesi, having children is a step towards ancestry (Kotilainen 1992:126).

18 *Sering kawin, 'nda pernah nikah.*

19 *Bakupiara* as translated by Babcock (1986:80).

20 Cf. Wikan (1990:5): 'a great many, perhaps most, marriages in North Bali are conducted by elopement (*merangkat*)...'.

21 On East Toraja, see Kotilainen (1992:117–26).

22 *Ibu*, 'Mrs', 'mother'. An Indonesian-language honorific and slightly formal title for a woman higher in status and/or than ego, who belongs in the 'middle', or parental, generation.

23 *Toto* means 'breast' or 'nipple' in Amurang.

24 This was so also in the beginning of the century (Gandhi-Lapian 1995:94).

25 In comparison, Rosemary Firth ([1943]1966:105–6) wrote about a child's position in a Malay fishing household that 25 per cent of children 'live outside normal simple family life'. They were either temporarily cared for by adults other than parents, adopted permanently,

looked after by widowed or divorced women or men, or looked after by a remarried parent. Of these, adoptions which were not legally sanctioned amounted to 11 per cent within the census area.

26 Contrary to Gandhi-Lapian (1995:101), according to *adat* law in old Minahasa an *anak piara*, despite being called *pahajoan*, did not have the status of a slave (Adatrechtbundel 1910 III:96–7). Although s/he had to work hard for a living in absence of any maintenance from the biological parents, there was a further reciprocal link with the new 'elders', as s/he could receive from them some inheritance after their death (ibid).

27 Some people equated 'big spirit' (*jiwa besar*) with 'high spiritedness' (*sumangat tinggi*), but Amurang fishermen's *sumangat* appears to be achieved rather than inherited.

28 His information comes from the Dutch missionary Warneck who worked in North Sulawesi.

29 According to the government's own announcement, 0.8 (maternal mortality) and 83 (infant mortality) per 1,000 live births in 1985 (Sarwono 1996:81).

CHAPTER 6

WOMEN, WORK AND PROCREATION BELIEFS IN TWO MUSLIM COMMUNITIES

ILDIKÓ BELLÉR-HANN

INTRODUCTION

In this paper I report on two recent fieldwork projects in relatively peripheral regions of the Muslim world. Among Lazi villagers in northeast Turkey my exploration of ideas concerning procreation started with the accidental discovery of an illuminating procreation metaphor. In more recent research among the Turkic-speaking Uighurs in the Chinese province of Xinjiang I was more consciously looking for beliefs concerning human procreation. In considering these issues I have found Carol Delaney's exploration and analysis of the 'seed and soil' metaphor of human procreation among Anatolian villagers inspiring (1986, 1991). Her villagers attribute the primary, active role in the creation of children to men as 'seed-givers', while women are relegated to a secondary, passive role as 'fields'. Delaney applies a hierarchically ordered monogenetic view of human procreation to virtually all details of social organization in an Anatolian village. She claims that this monogenetic view of procreation is linked to monotheistic religions and presents one large tidy system of beliefs. In her words:

> paternity is embedded in an entire matrix of beliefs about the world and the way it is constructed.... From the most intimate to ultimate contexts, from physical to metaphysical realities, an entire world is constructed and systematically interrelated. (1986:510).

Leela Dube's study of the symbolism of biological reproduction in India complements that of Delaney and pays special attention to the correspondence between procreation ideology and the ideologies and realities of women's role in agricultural production. She argues that

> man's rights over the woman do not relate only to her sexuality and reproductive capacity, but encompass her productive capacities and labour power also. Just as he is entitled to have control over her sexuality and over the product of her sexuality, he is entitled to have control over her labour and also the proceeds of her labour. (Dube 1986:43–4).

From this Dube concludes that women's role in cultivation is devalued to a merely supportive role and that the under-recognition of women's economic contribution matches the asymmetrical ideology of human procreation. The unequal contribution of the two sexes to human reproduction, as expressed through the symbolism of 'seed and earth', provides the rationalization for a system in which women stand alienated from productive resources, have no control over their own labour power, and are denied rights over their offspring (Dube 1986). Similar conclusions about labour are reached in the north Indian context by Jeffery and Jeffery, who point out that 'women's work is … trivialized and brings them little credit' (1993:12).

My findings in two Muslim communities show that procreation beliefs similar to the 'seed and soil metaphor' are sometimes articulated in modified forms, tailored to local conditions, while at other times, although encapsulated in language itself, they are never given full conscious expression. I shall argue that, as Dube suggests, there is indeed a correspondence between procreation beliefs and the evaluation of women's participation in production, but that these two domains do not always parallel each other. In the case of the Lazi a well-articulated procreation metaphor shows women as subordinate and passive in human procreation, but at the same time it implicitly recognizes women's role as primary agricultural producers. Among the Uighurs 'seed and soil' type procreation ideas are implicit in kinship vocabulary and some commonly held beliefs, but contemporary informants may not have explicit knowledge of the metaphor. Within a patriarchal setting, man and woman are here attributed an equal role in the making of a child, but this symmetry accompanies a conspicuous underplaying of women's role as economic producers. The two cases lead us to the tentative conclusion that ideological recognition of women's productive or reproductive roles may be linked to variations in social organization, such as a new migration pattern or changed assumptions about the nature of marriage. In such situations it is as if the necessity to maintain the ideological fiction of male supremacy required the accentuation of gender asymmetry in at least one of the two domains.

BASKETS AMONG THE LAZI

Among both the Lazi and the Uighurs information was collected from several villages in quite separate locations rather than from one small, bounded community. Both groups have been settled agriculturalists for a long time, albeit in very different natural environments, and both are characterized by patriarchy and virilocal residence patterns. Both are Sunni Muslims, and form ethnically and linguistically small minorities in states dominated by very much larger ethnic/linguistic majorities, though in the case of the Lazi they are not differentiated from the majority by religion. A group of Caucasian origin, the Lazi occupy a strip of the Black Sea coast in the northeastern corner of Turkey.[1] Although they were converted to Islam about four hundred years ago, their pre-Islamic, Christian past has been completely erased from their collective memory. Their strong identification with Islam is a reflection of their high level of integration into the Turkish state, although many Lazi have retained their original Caucasian language. Their distinctive accents and a number of stereotypical characteristics mark them out when away from home. The biggest change within living memory was the introduction of tea as a cash crop in the mid-1950s, which quickly replaced what had been predominantly a subsistence economy.[2]

The Lazi region borders on the district of Of, where the American anthropologist Michael Meeker carried out fieldwork in the 1970s. An important ethnographic detail in Delaney's seed-and soil argument, in fact the strongest factual support for her theory, is actually quoted from Meeker's fieldwork:

> If you plant wheat, you get wheat. If you plant barley, you get barley. It is the seed which determines the kind of plant which will grow, while the field nourishes the plant but does not

determine the kind. The man gives the seed, and the woman is like the field. (Meeker 1970:157; quoted in Delaney 1986:497).

During many conversations with Lazi, Turkish and Hemşinli[3] men and women in the region I came across a metaphor which likens women not to a field but to a basket. Lazi women are closely associated with the carrying of baskets and other weights. This is often one of the first points people make when evaluating women's position in this region. Although many locals are eager to point out that the lot of the Lazi woman has improved dramatically in recent decades, they also agree that the number of women to be seen carrying heavy weights along paths and roads far outstrips the number of men.

Baskets and material culture

Basket-making has a long tradition among the Lazi. The four main types have been described as unique to the Lazi by Feurstein (1983:53–60) who considers two types, *kalati* and *tikina*, a kind of 'ethnic marker' (p. 56).[4] These baskets have been described by Turkish folklorists as 'the ingenious invention of the people of the Eastern Black Sea coast', and as an inseparable part of women's life in this region.[5] The stereotype of the Lazi woman, well known throughout the rest of Turkey, depicts her carrying an enormous loaded basket on her back. Young girls start carrying a miniature version at an early age.

Baskets are an adaptation to the geographical conditions of the traditional Lazi settlements, which are scattered steep valleys where narrow mountain paths limited transportation options until very recent times. Women in their seventies recall how in their youth, before the introduction of tea, they used to go to market carrying their produce in their baskets, which were then filled with shopping for the return journey. Feurstein in his excellent work on the material culture of the Lazi notes that the largest basket has associations with human living quarters. In the Fndkl Lazuri dialect the word means a 'woven hut' and he points out that the shape of this basket is that of a round hut turned upside down. Furthermore, he adds, this large basket was exclusively carried by women, and it was mainly employed for carrying grass in mountain villages, where animal husbandry was of particular importance (Feurstesin 1983:55).

As far as the *tikina* and the *kalati* are concerned, Feurstein draws a parallel between baskets and humans on the basis that these baskets have little 'feet'. This parallel seems to be confirmed by the fact that in Georgian, to which Lazuri is closely related, the word *iina*, itself a derivative of *tikina kalati*, also means 'baby' (Feurstein 1983:58). In the past large baskets were used for carrying ferns, leaves and hay and the smaller type for collecting fruit (ibid.: 1983:54). Nowadays baskets are still used for carrying tea, wood, grass/fodder for the animals, and shopping. Although most villages now have at least a basic single-track dirt road, Lazi women still frequently carry heavy burdens on their backs in baskets.

Baskets and symbolic culture

Most informants, regardless of ethnic affiliation, are also familiar with the basket as symbol and metaphor and associate it with the Lazi. The metaphor exists in several versions in the Lazuri language.[6] Usually Lazi men were thoroughly embarrassed when asked about it, but Lazi women's reaction was – most of the time – a hearty laughter.

In Pazar and Ardeşen, the two western, more conservative districts of the Lazi region, the metaphor sounds something like this: 'A woman is a basket: you empty it and then fill it again.' (Turkish: *Kadn sepettur. Boş*altyorsun, sonra yine dolduruyorsun).[7] I first heard this metaphor from a 25-year-old village girl, who was telling me about her own difficult position. She had been proposed to by a young man from another Lazi village, and although she knew that she should accept because she had reached the age beyond which she would be regarded as a spinster whose fate was 'closed' (T. *ksmeti kapanmş*), she nevertheless declined. Her main reason was that she did not want to carry on living in a village, not even married to a good husband.

> The work is too hard here for women. And then they have to give birth to many children and they are ruined in no time. Women here age quickly. But what shall we do? A woman is a basket, and her fate is to be filled and emptied again.

She said this with a grave face.[8] Her use of the metaphor brought together two of the most important aspects of women's life: biological reproduction and economic production.[9] After this incidental discovery of the metaphor I began to ask about baskets more systematically in and around ethnically mixed Pazar. All women who were familiar with it agreed that it was a Lazi metaphor which the Hemşinli and ethnic Turks did not endorse: it was said to be an expression of Lazi women's degraded position. Lazi villagers usually stated that the 'basket metaphor' emphasized two aspects of women's life: their heavy workload and their reproductive function. A full basket is like a pregnant woman, an empty one like a woman before getting pregnant, after giving birth or between two pregnancies. Alternatively, an empty basket may also stand for barrenness. An empty basket is seen as one which can and should be filled. Just as the purpose of a basket is to be filled, the function of a woman is to reproduce. This idea is consistent with the underlying Islamic view that children are a gift of God, and that getting married and having children is the only acceptable course of life.

Some interpretations of the basket metaphor appeared to emphasize the passive role of the Lazi woman in reproduction. She is said to be the mere recipient of others' (men's) actions: the filling is under the exclusive control of the male. I was told that one can, if one wishes, dispose of a basket if it proves to be useless, replacing it with a better one. One woman unambiguously voiced the fears of many: 'A woman is a basket. You throw the old one away and replace it with a new one.' (Turkish: *Kadn sepettur. Eskisini atarsn, yenisini alrsn.*) A woman who stays empty for too long (a sign of barrenness) can be sent back to her father's home and another woman found in her place. Most people agree that the most frequent reason for a second, polygamous marriage is the first wife's inability to produce a male heir. This kind of interpretation, though often stated in humorous fashion by the villagers themselves, is no joke at all. Male offspring are a must and women have to keep trying for a son, even after the birth of as many as seven or eight daughters. Divorce cases are often initiated as a result of the woman's alleged barrenness or her 'inability' to produce a son. Divorcees, especially those whose previous marriage was childless, find it hard to remarry and have lower social status in their fathers' or brothers' household, where they return after divorce, than married mothers and widows. The stigma of barrenness is exclusively carried by the woman. Although under social pressure to become mothers and to produce sons, Lazi women are painfully aware that bearing many children and their heavy workload combine to affect their health and beauty. They often say that they age quickly and that this, too, may cause them to lose their men to other, younger women.

Informants explain the basket metaphor in terms which point to a complete lack of agency for women, in a context of virilocal residence patterns and the basically temporary nature of their stay with their natal family. In contrast to women, who are temporary and potentially ready to move on or rather to be moved on, men are seen as permanent. This idea is expressed in a simile, which was told to me by Lazi girls when interpreting the basket metaphor: 'A man is like a lake, a woman is like a stream.' (Turkish: *Erkek göl gibi, kadn dere gibi.*) In spite of this representation of women as temporary, in a community where long-term labour migration has become part and parcel of many families' lives the incoming women may yet come to be more settled and permanent in their husbands' homes than the men themselves. This attitude may be detected when women give an account of the size of a household: they usually start by counting the number of brides (T. *gelin*).

A variation of the 'seed and soil' metaphor can also be heard among the Lazi: 'Whatever you sow will grow.' (Turkish: *Ne ekersen, o biter.*) The explanation may continue: 'if you plant cabbages, you grow cabbages and not carrots'. This saying can be conflated with the basket metaphor to result in something like: 'whatever you put into the basket is what will come out of it'. I only ever heard the pure 'seed and soil' metaphor explicitly mentioned by one Lazi, a man of exceptional knowledge himself engaged in local ethnographic research: 'A woman is like a field, whatever you sow will grow'. (Turkish: *Kadn tarlaya benzer. Ne ekersen o biter*. Lazuri: *Oxorca ontules nugams. Mu xackare heya yulun.*) A very similar proverb was repeatedly quoted by villagers: 'a nettle produces a nettle', (Turkish: *Isrgan otu srgan otu yapar*. Lazuri: *Tutucik tuci eligams.*) The popularity of such sayings suggests that the Lazi, like Delaney's (1991) villagers elsewhere in Anatolia, and those close by studied by Meeker (1970), believe that men play the predominant role in human procreation. Informants readily confirm the gender asymmetry which gets articulated in the basket metaphor. One young, educated government clerk claimed that 75 per cent of a child's characteristics are determined by the father.

The carrying of heavy weights also figures in speech about female bodily functions. Because of the lack of sex education, either at home or at school, young village girls are often taken by surprise at the onset of menarche and attribute it to their having carried heavy weights. People also say that it is easy for a woman to resume work after she has given birth, because she has been relieved of her heavy load. A local midwife related that miscarriage during the early stages of pregnancy used to be prevented by tying belts around the woman's abdomen to stop the baby from 'falling' (Turkish: *düşmesin*), in the same way as heavy weights may be tied to a woman's back to prevent them from falling off.

Reproduction, patriarchy and the value of work

The basket metaphor may be less widespread than the metaphors discussed by Delaney (1991) and Dube (1986), and possibly the exclusive property of a region in which the geography has dictated the use of baskets in shifting goods. I think it is significant that in this metaphor, which draws attention to women's central role in production, it is their reproductive function rather than their sexuality that gets the major emphasis, which contrasts with Delaney's account (1991:97). The basket metaphor is often quoted in connection with mothers: 'The mother is a basket. She has emptied.' (Lazuri: *Nana alation. Mocodinu.*) This emphasis may also be noticed in a Black Sea joke giving the definition of woman, which I was told by a man from the district of Ardeşen: 'A man from the Black Sea is asked "What is a woman?" "A woman is someone with a baby on her lap,".he answers.'[10] (*T. Karadenizliden sorarlar: 'Kadn nedir?' 'Kucağnda bebektir.'*) Commenting on the basket metaphor informants also said that it expressed the idea that a woman is a tool, both for work and for childbearing, and that she has no value in herself.

The strong association of baskets and women's reproductive functions is clarified in the gender specificity of basket carrying. Feurstein states that Lazi men have traditionally refused to carry baskets (1983:36). A local solicitor told me that when he was a student on holiday he once tried to help out in his village by carrying a heavy basket. His female relatives were appalled and objected by saying that his behaviour was shameful (*ayp*), and it would be *their* shame if their men were seen performing such a task. When pressed for an explanation of this attitude on the women's part, some women rationalized it in relation to the long-term migration that has prevailed among the Lazi for a long time. Since at least the nineteenth century, many Lazi men went to Russia to work as long-term migrant labourers to escape poverty, a trend which has continued in the Republican period, though its direction has largely shifted to the big cities of Turkey, Germany and Saudi Arabia (Marr 1910:618; Toumarkine 1995:85). During men's absence women have had to manage farms alone. Not only has male labour migration remained an important component of the local economy, but the cultivation of tea from the 1950s has become primarily identified as female work. Women say that since their men are often absent for longer periods of time and work hard for their families, it would be unfair to make them perform hard work when they come back. Some men say that it is this attitude on the women's part which has made them spoilt, and less likely to offer help with carrying. Today it is possible to see men with baskets on their backs, but often these are Kurdish sharecroppers or ethnic Turks from neighbouring regions, who are unfamiliar with the local gender associations of the basket.

The social context within which the basket metaphor has become articulated is characterized by stable marriages and very low divorce rates. Polygamy, though illegal in the state's eyes, is still practised but is becoming increasingly rare. But great emphasis is laid upon women's conformity to the modesty code and community sanctions for women and men who do not conform are harsh. The great importance placed on virginity at marriage[11] and the relatively low status of divorcees upon return to their natal home are part of a pattern which values women's chastity and guarantees paternity rights in circumstances where husbands are often absent through long-term labour migration. In cases of divorce, local custom asserts the father's right to his children. Nowadays children may remain with the mother, who may have little choice but to retreat into her natal home.[12] Control over the product of female labour is usually in male hands, if men are present at all, although there are significant variations in this respect between the different valleys. Overall this can reasonably be labelled a patriarchal society.

If a child turns out to be particularly difficult, or perhaps retarded, it is the mother's side which gets the blame. It is said that 'the child takes after his maternal uncle' (Turkish: *Çocuk daydan çeker, sen daydan bozuksun*). This is clearly a way of putting the blame on the woman, or at least on her side, while at the same time reinforcing man's primary role in procreation.[13] In reality the woman herself does get victimized by her husband when children turn out badly. The maternal uncle (Turkish: *day*) is meticulously distinguished from the paternal uncle (*amca*) in Turkish, and the same Turkish designations are used in Lazuri, too. In a rapidly disappearing part of the local wedding ceremony, when the groom and his party go to fetch the bride, sums of money are requested by her family for 'milk right' (Turkish: *süt hakk*, payable to the mother), 'brother's right' (Turkish: *kardeş* hakk, payable to one of the girl's brothers) and 'maternal uncle's right' (Turkish: *day hakk*). Explanations of this custom turn on the exceptional proximity of the maternal uncle to his sister and through her to her children. They are from the same womb, and he therefore has special responsibilities towards his sister's family. The paternal uncle is not considered close enough to have the same rights.

Controversy concerning the biological proximity of the paternal and maternal uncles finds expression in local definitions of the modesty code articulated in the concept of *namahram*.[14] The term, which is widely used to govern women's everyday behaviour in relation to men, separates all men from the female ego's point of view into those covered by the incest taboo with whom therefore a woman can be more intimate, and those who are not covered by the taboo, and therefore potential marriage partners for her: in the presence of all those who fall into this latter category, referred to as *namahram* (literally a canonical stranger), a woman must at all times maintain spatial distance and observe the rules of modesty such as keeping her hair, arms and legs fully covered, etc. With non-*namahram* males such as her father, son, brother, etc. a woman is free to relax the modesty rules, since marriage/sexual relations are strongly prohibited between her and him.[15] About half of those asked considered that the maternal uncle (*day*) was so close to a woman that he could not be considered *namahram* (i.e. a canonical stranger) to her, because he and her mother had come from the same womb, while everyone maintained that the paternal uncle was *namahram*. Others argued that both were *namahram* and therefore there was no difference in proximity between them as regards their niece.

These beliefs deviate from the Koranic view, which makes no distinction between the maternal and the paternal uncles. They would seem to go against the bias in favour of the male side, as expressed in the 'seed and soil' theory. However, ideas surrounding first cousin marriage reinforce it. First cousin marriages are said to have been common in this region for a long time and even today, despite large-scale government campaigns, the practice continues. Most informants agree that ideal marriage partners from the point of view of the male ego listed in order of biological proximity include: 1. FBD (*amca kz*) 2. MBD (*day kz*) 3. FZD (*hala kz*) 4. MZD (*teyze kz*) There is general consensus that two brothers' children are the most closely related (through the father's blood), while the biological link between two sisters is the loosest.[16] The contradiction in these examples, between the proximity created by the maternal link in some instances and the priority given to the paternal side in others, is more apparent than real. As Dube has pointed out for India, the mother's contribution can be recognized and emphasized in the moral context of obligations, while the father's contribution is nonetheless articulated in terms of his right over the child (Dube 1986:36). The somewhat enigmatic role of the Lazi maternal uncle may similarly be seen as an expression of the moral obligation transmitted by the female line.

In everyday life the basket as an implement is mainly associated with women's work. In the metaphor the woman becomes what in daily life she is most closely and visibly associated with during her outdoor activities. There is a clear visual parallel between carrying a heavy basket and being pregnant and the walk of a pregnant woman is not unlike the walk of someone carrying a large load on her back. Local newspapers actively promote the stereotype of the basket-carrying Lazi woman as a symbol of the eastern Black Sea coast. In contrast to Delaney's (1991) observations, work has enormous prestige in the Lazi region, both for the Lazi and for neighbouring ethnic groups.[17] The ability to carry heavy loads enhances the attractions of a girl as a potential wife, and is a source of pride among women, just like pregnancy. The implication is that whoever is capable of carrying heavy loads is strong and healthy, someone who will also be capable of coping with numerous pregnancies. In opposition to the commonly held Islamic idea that women are weak and vulnerable, the image and self-perception of Lazi women show them as strong agents, who are capable of heavy work and of looking after the household economy during their husbands' absences.

We may therefore interpret the basket metaphor in two very different ways. It is an encapsulation of women's subordinate position, passivity, lack of agency, substitutability. For many informants the metaphor is also an assertion of women's primary role as workers and agricultural producers. The attribution of lack of agency is valid enough as far as human reproduction is concerned, but women as producers and labourers have an extremely positive image in the whole eastern Black Sea region, and their self-perceptions underline this. 'There is no work in the village that a woman does not do,' said one young Lazi girl. In the absence of historical sources it is impossible to tell whether the basket metaphor and the meanings associated with it emerged as a result of large-scale migration, or whether the present combination of elements has even older roots in Lazi culture.

THE UIGHURS: NO METAPHOR, NO ASYMMETRY?

My second set of data comes from more recent fieldwork in northwest China among the Turkic-speaking Uighurs.[18] The Uighurs changed from a nomadic way of life to a settled agricultural economy over a thousand years ago. Their ancestors had embraced a variety of world views and religions before they were converted to Islam, probably in the sixteenth century. Perhaps the most dramatic changes in Uighur peasants' lives started in 1949 with the 'Liberation' which marked the beginning of Chinese communist rule. This was soon followed by the collectivization of agriculture, which persisted until the early 1980s. Since then, in another dramatic turn, economic reform and decollectivization have once again transformed life in the countryside.[19]

The 'seed' of a metaphor

I shall discuss procreation beliefs in the context of two sets of ideas, the first reflecting Islamic ontology, the second consisting of folk theories focused on the human body. Various sources make references to God's creation from clay/earth of the first man, the Prophet Adam, who then married Eve, the first woman (Katanov and Menges [1933]1976:1206–7; Häbibulla 1993:389;

Raxman et al.1996:172). But even the mythical beginnings of humankind are not entirely free of bodily images. A story (*hikayä*) collected by Jarring from a farmer and *mollah* in 1935 focuses on the bodily aspects of sexual intercourse between the first couple. The description, an example of the intermingling of the sacred and the profane, makes no use of metaphor and instead of human procreation focuses on a miracle, the creation of the jade stone:

> The holy Adam – peace be upon him – and mother Eve were separated from each other for seven years. One day the holy Adam – peace be upon him – and mother Eve met each other on a glacier.... They had coition at this place. The seminal fluid flowed out on the glacier. The seminal fluid froze. From this the jade stone has its origin. That is the miracle of the holy Adam – peace be upon him. That women feel cold on their rump and men on their knees has remained from this time. (Jarring 1951:III 64).

Metaphors are also absent from other native descriptions of birth and connected practices. In an essay dating from the 1930s Muhammad Ali Damollah describes the power of God by saying that humans 'pass from the loins of the father to the womb of the mother. When at a certain period of time they receive soul [*jan*] their mother's menstruation stops and (the baby) feeds on the mother's blood. (*Prov.207.I*: 22).[20]

I found that contemporary informants also had no explicit knowledge of a procreation metaphor comparable to the basket metaphor or that of the seed and the soil. However, language and some beliefs surrounding procreation point to an implicit familiarity with the seed and soil beliefs. The word for seminal fluid used by the storyteller quoted by Jarring above is *mäni*, which is associated by informants primarily with male blood. Synonymous with this is *uruq*, which also means 'seed' and 'species' (Schwarz 1992:582,894). The generic word for 'relative' is *uruq-tuqqan*, the first element meaning seed, and the second a past participle derived from the verb '*tuğ* – to give birth to, to lay eggs, to bear fruit (*bala tuğ* – 'to give birth to a child'; *tuxum tuğ* – 'to lay an egg') (ibid.: 226). However, even older people could not elaborate on such clues encoded in the language.[21] One elderly woman said that a new-born baby is like the growing wheat plant which never grows alone but is always surrounded by plants of a similar sort, thereby emphasizing the social aspect of birth: human beings are surrounded by relatives from the second they are born. In spite of thirty years of socialist collectivization, the old belief that women should not go to the fields because 'if they were to go, so would fertility' is still well remembered, although rarely adhered to literally. However, the rule that under no circumstances should women sow the seeds of wheat or corn is rigorously observed. The association of the sowing of grain seed exclusively with men may be seen as another implicit manifestation of the seed and soil beliefs.

The term *uruq-tuqqan* means all types of relatives, both maternal and paternal. Another term, *qandaş* (derived from *qan* = 'blood'; *-daş* = a suffix expressing companionship) is also used to denote close relatives, relatives related by blood. The term *qerindaş* (derived from *qarin* = 'belly, stomach') is usually used in conjunction with *qandaş* in the form *qan-qerindaş*, the dictionary meaning of which is given as 'blood brother' (Schwarz 1992:627). The main substance provided by the mother to the child is milk (*süt*) while the father contributes blood (*qan*). The quotation above from Muhammad Ali Damollah indicates that during pregnancy the baby is supposed to feed on its mother's blood and milk, as female substance becomes prominent only after the birth. But milk and the womb remain intimately connected in the popular imagination: milk siblings (*emildaş*), though otherwise unrelated, are considered to be 'of the same womb' (*qerindaş*), and in line with Quranic edict are prohibited from marrying. One informant insisted that *qandaş* means those of the same blood, i.e. children of two full brothers, while *qerindaş* (those of the same womb) stands for the children of two sisters. Most, however, maintained that *qandaş* are all those sharing a father, *qerindaş* are children sharing a mother, and *qan-qerindaş* originally referred to full siblings by the same father and mother. Children of the same father are said to share the same blood group.

This explanation makes sense within the given social context. For at least the past hundred years there has been a very high incidence of divorce and remarriage among the Uighurs.[22] Unlike the situation described by Dube (1986:42) and many other Muslim societies, among the Uighurs for a woman to leave her children with their biological father and to remarry while they are young is not considered shameful but normal practice. 'Social ownership' of the child has customarily been assigned to the father's side. It is also the father's side which exercises the right to choose a name for the new-born. Giving up their children is usually interpreted by women as a practice which is necessary for them to be able to remarry. Distinguishing between siblings who shared a father but not a mother and those who shared a mother but not a father was important in determining rights over children and property. As among the Lazi, entitlement to property through inheritance in customary law reveals gender asymmetry. In accordance with Islamic values women are regarded as lawful heirs of their biological father's property but their share is supposed to be half or less than that of their brothers (*Prov.464*:40v; *Prov.207.I*:5). In practice land is usually divided among male heirs only and women inherit land only if they have no brothers.[23]

A symmetrical model of biological procreation

Although one may be implicitly found in the language and some social practices, neither historical nor contemporary sources reveal a fully developed procreation metaphor of seed and the soil, although alternative metaphoric allusions to sexual relations are not unknown. Jarring gives the following indigenous description of a Muslim shrine (*mazar*) at Yarkand. 'Every Sunday a number of women go to that shrine [saying] 'Oh, ghodja of the shrine! Give me a husband who can take care of his house! Give me a man who can put a ladle into the kettle' ... thus they pray crying' (Jarring 1951:IV 174). Jarring notes that 'the women are praying for children: 'ladle' and 'kettle' probably allude to the sexual organs of man and woman'. This description of women's prayers at the shrine of a female saint corresponds closely to another informant's account of this same ritual, also practised by childless women wishing for a child.

> Unmarried women made a cooking pot out of two pieces of clay, put two more pieces of clay, firewood and some bran in it. This meant that they asked 'we have put up a pot, we have put a ladle in it – we wish for a good husband, lord of the shrine'. (Tenishev 1984:65–6).[24]

Both references concern the shrine of the saint known as Süt Padişahim or 'Lady Milk' (cf. Baldick 1993:191–2). Milk is, of course, the female substance *per se*. However, it is hard to tell to what an extent such a form of prayer was widespread or known outside Yarkand.

In contrast to the gender asymmetry implicit in the seed and soil and the basket metaphor, data from Xinjiang support a binary, symmetrical model of procreation. Some informants say that the child may look like his mother, but usually inherits his father's humoral disposition (*mijäz*).[25] Most agree that, like the sex of the unborn child, this too depends upon God's will (although several informants claimed that the sex of the child depends on the degree of love and passion between the parents at the time of conception).[26]

Getting married and having children is regarded as the most desirable course of life for a woman. Women who cannot conceive resort to a variety of practices to ensure pregnancy. Barrenness is sometimes blamed on the woman, but more often it is acknowledged that either party can be at fault. A divorcee is not stigmatized and even if her previous marriage was childless she can remarry without difficulty.[27] Informants confirm that young divorcees who have already had children from a previous marriage are often considered more desirable marriage partners than unmarried girls.[28]

Some beliefs surrounding menstruation and childbearing attribute positive outcomes (the birth of a beautiful child) to the workings of the female body, while negative outcomes may be blamed on male action. Menstruation (*häyiz*, *adät*, *xun*) is considered an illness *(käsäl)*. Some rural women insist that this is the way women's bodies are regularly cleansed of their sins because, as men and women agree, women have a great many sins by nature. Although the absence of menstruation is often a sign of pregnancy, they also know of cases when women continue to bleed during pregnancy. If this is the case the woman is likely to have a particularly beautiful child, since her body keeps on purifying itself. Menstruation is a state of pollution during which time no sexual intercourse should take place between man and wife. But some men do break the prohibition, and children conceived during this time are said to be deformed as a result of God's punishment.[29]

Kinship terminology makes no distinction between the maternal and paternal uncles (both are called *tağa*) or maternal and paternal aunts (both are called *hamma*). Close-kin marriages have been prevalent despite a government ban, but informants do not differentiate degrees of proximity between the various possibilities on the paternal and maternal sides. Qing images of the peoples of Xinjiang dating from the second half of the eighteenth century also noted that among the Turkis (today known as Uighurs) a man's children by various wives were considered of equal rank (apart from birth order seniority), and a woman's children by different husbands were regarded as consanguineous (Millward 1993:266).

In addition to an egalitarian, symmetrical view of procreation some persistent traditions emphasize the close links maintained through the female line, and the celebration of fertility. Villagers say that at least the first two children must be born in the woman's natal house with her mother's assistance, though subsequent births may take place at the husband's house. This tradition persists today in rural areas and even among urban intellectuals. Rural women express their preference for giving birth in their natal home by saying that their own mothers are the best ones to look after them; ideally they would like to return home for each subsequent birth, but their husband may not give consent after the second occasion. This practice is described as common 'in societies where marriages tend to be unstable, where there is not a great deal of trust and cooperation between husband and wife, or where the matrifocal family is common' (MacCormack 1982:13).

Textual material from the first half of this century reveals that when a baby was born to a middle income or rich family, they called together the midwives (*toğutçi xotun, toğut anisi*) to help with the birth. As soon as the baby was born his/her umbilical cord (*kindik*) had to be cut by a close female relative of the mother, such as her grandmother or her mother or any other woman with a good disposition (*xuy*) and morality (*äxlaq*). It was thought that the child's temper and habits will be similar to those of this person; in other words, a woman is held responsible for the qualities of a child (*Prov.212*:2–3). *Toğut anisi* was synonymous with the term *kindik anisi* (the mother of the umbilical cord) which implies that the cutting of the cord was often done by the midwife herself. Contemporary informants confirm that after the birth the placenta, (*äş* or *yoldaş*) must be buried in the mud floor of the house. If this is not done the baby will be unlucky, may become sick or even die (*Prov.207.II.*12:1). Rumour has it that, following deliveries in modern hospitals, only the male child's placenta is preserved to be used for making medicine. Women assume that female babies' placentas are thrown away as rubbish, and some are extremely unhappy about this. However, this equal concern for babies is not necessarily reflected in all areas of childcare: female children are usually breastfed for shorter periods of time than male children, and the birth of a male child was said to be celebrated more elaborately in the past (*Prov.212*:7). However, some informants confirm that the 'cradle ritual', a large celebration, is more likely to be organized for a girl than for a boy. It is viewed by some as a 'compensation' for girls since each brother will have celebrations following circumcision.

Before 'Liberation' in 1949 which marked the incorporation of the province of Xinjiang into communist China, a common practice among well-to-do and rich families was the 'hair-tying ritual' (*çaçwaq toyi, çaç qoş*aq) or 'ritual of the young married woman' *(juwan toyi*).[30] Informants say that this ritual was always organized in the woman's parents' home, either during her first or later pregnancy, or shortly after she has given birth to her first or second baby. Since the first few births invariably took place in the woman's natal home, the celebration too was held there. It involved a great many presents for the woman from her natal family, from her husband and from his family. Her hairstyle was permanently changed, and minor alterations were made to the ornamentation of her dress. These changes marked her transition from the status of *çokan* (young married woman without children) to the status of *juwan* (young married woman with children). That this was a rite of passage for the woman (sometimes described as grander and more important than the actual wedding) and not a celebration of the baby is clear from the fact that this ritual could only be performed once in a woman's lifetime; it could not be repeated, even if none of her babies survived. Although this practice was apparently restricted to the well-to-do classes, informants and earlier records suggest that this celebration was an ideal for other families as well.

Relationships with the mother and through the female side are very important among contemporary Uighurs. Rudelson (1997:126) describes how in Urumchi, the provincial capital of the Xinjiang Uighur Autonomous Region, he found that young married couples maintained closest ties with the wife's sister and her husband; these were much closer than, for example, ties between couples related by two brothers. One explanation for the phenomenon may be the prevalence of avoidance rules between males. A young man feels more relaxed (e.g. he can smoke and drink) in the company of his wife's sister's husband than in the presence of his elder brothers.

The devaluing of women's work

The relative freedom and power of women in this region in comparison with adjacent Muslim lands was remarked upon by many travellers in the nineteenth and early twentieth centuries as well as by Chinese sources (Warikoo 1985; Mackerras 1995:78). Grenard goes to great lengths to elaborate on the historical antecedents of such practices, which he connects to social customs rooted in pre-Islamic times (Grenard 1898:123–4). Although such antecedents remain speculative, they cannot be dismissed as completely without foundation. The brand of Islam developed in Xinjiang has allowed women to give birth in their natal home, the fertility ritual of 'hair-tying', frequent divorce and a symmetrical explanation of procreation. Women's reproductive role has thus been given enormous emphasis. However, in contrast to the Lazi, Uighur women's contribution to production seems to have been consistently played down. Since pre-'Liberation' times women have been regarded as weak and vulnerable (*ajiz*). Their activities are ideally restricted to the home: rural women are not associated with cash earning.[31] Old people sometimes assert that before 1949 no woman worked in the fields because of the modesty code expressed in the concept of *namahram*. Closer questioning reveals that this was an ideal rather than an absolute rule, and that poorer women did work in the fields. As in other peasant societies, Uighur women's participation in agricultural work depended on their social standing and showed a great deal of variation. But the value system prevailing before 1949 saw women as home-makers and mothers rather than as agricultural producers. This state of affairs changed drastically after 'Liberation', when women became active contributors to agricultural production and the working woman was vigorously promoted by the State (Davin 1976; Croll 1979). The thirty years between 1950 and 1980, the time of economic reforms, were extremely disruptive in every aspect of Uighur villagers' lives. While officials today like to maintain that it was during this period that Uighur women became liberated from the yoke of patriarchy, the villagers' own accounts of those times tell a different story. By ordering women into the fields the communist authorities violated the rule of *namahram* and flouted traditional norms, if not necessarily traditional practice.

Since the economic reforms of the early 1980s the old value system seems to have been revived among Uighur villagers, though with important modifications. A woman's place is seen once more as being in the home. Although some deny that *namahram* rules still apply, in practice most women do observe them in everyday life. But women are visibly present in the fields. As in the past, they play the primary role in cotton production. They work alongside men in the wheat and corn fields. All this work outside the home is described as 'helping their husbands'. In households where animal husbandry is the major source of cash income, the women who are responsible for virtually all the work involved describe it as part of their household chores, while husbands get public recognition for such work. In one hamlet where many women take a large share in felt-making, the major source of household income, the women describe themselves as having 'no special skills', as merely 'helping' their husbands. The men, in contrast, are perceived as skilled felt-makers. Women who engage in embroidering and marketing hats (*doppa*) maintain that this is a leisure activity, even when it takes up to five or six hours a day.

CONCLUSION

The two peoples discussed in this chapter both belong to regions which have been characterized in terms of their dominant agricultural practices as male farming systems (Boserup 1970), illustrating the Eurasian model of plough agriculture (Goody 1976), and have been associated with hierarchical social systems and relatively restricted roles for women (Jeffery and Jeffery 1993:8). However, in spite of the differences in climate and surroundings, the traditional, largely subsistence economies of both the Lazi and the Uighurs were in fact hoe-based. The plough, though known to both groups, was never adopted by either, which may explain why an artefact prominent in the seed and soil beliefs depicted by Dube and Delaney does not figure in the procreation beliefs of these people (Dube 1986:41; Delaney 1991:49). Among the Lazi, baskets, the implements primarily associated with women, are considered the symbol of agricultural work. In contrast, among the Uighurs it is the hoe (*kätmän*), associated with male work, which has achieved this symbolic status.[32] But both sets of data exhibit important elements of the monogenetic theory of procreation, although neither is without complications and contradictions. This is only to be expected once we accept that there is no such thing as a static, fully developed Islamic world view. Local ideas and traditions, the uneven penetration of western scientific thought and the State, contacts with other ethnic groups, and the pace of modernization must all be considered. The data presented here suggest that there is a close relationship between ideas about women's presumed participation in biological reproduction and their perceived role in production. Among the Lazi, women's primary role in agricultural production is publicly recognized, but their role in reproduction is played down. These two aspects of women's roles are expressed in the 'basket metaphor'. A woman's pregnancy and subordination to men have been likened to her most conspicuous work, carrying. The Uighurs are similarly a patriarchal society and women's reproductive function has traditionally been emphasized. Here the seed and soil metaphor, though present in traces, is overshadowed by a more balanced idea of human reproduction. However, women's considerable economic role has been devalued, and this has not changed in spite of the drastic changes enforced by the communist government over the past 40 years.

These two Muslim communities, remote from each other, have had very different social, political and economic histories. The monogenetic theory identified by Delaney as shaping decisively the overarching world view of peoples with monotheistic religions is admirably clear in her account, but hardly borne out by other ethnographic realities. Real communities have never existed in isolation, free of changes from internal and external sources, imposing the same views on all community members. The social context may in some places evoke fully elaborated metaphors, while in other circumstances these remain latent. Patriarchy can be maintained regardless of the extent to which women's role in production or biological reproduction is recognized. I suggest that in such cases, even if there is positive recognition of the role of women in one domain, their role in the other domain tends to be negated or underrepresented.

ACKNOWLEDGEMENTS

This paper is the outcome of fieldwork carried out jointly with Chris Hann supported by two grants from the Economic and Social Research Council of Great Britain R00023 3208 01 (1991–1993) and R00023 5709 (1994–1997). My thanks are primarily due to the Turkish and Chinese authorities, to Professor Tsui Yen Hu and Professor Fang Xiaohua, who were instrumental in obtaining a research permit in China, and to a great many individuals in the research areas. Ambassador Gunnar Jarring has been generous in allowing me unlimited access to his unpublished materials and with many helpful comments. Wolfgang Feurstein and James Millward have kindly given me permission to quote from their dissertations. Finally, I am indebted to Peter Loizos and Patrick Heady, for their many useful comments and suggestions.

NOTES

1 The term 'Laz' as an ethnic marker is highly ambiguous. In general it is used to designate regional identity, in which sense it covers all the coastal people living east of Samsun, most of whom today, regardless of their ethnogenetic history, are monolingual Turkic speakers. Even in this broad sense the term is a shifting one. Only a small group in the far eastern corner of Turkey's Black Sea region who today number approximately 200,000 people identify themselves as 'real' Laz. In addition to Turkish they speak their own, Caucasian language called Lazuri. Since my data were collected among the Lazuri speakers, to distinguish them from the wider category of Laz I shall refer to them as the Lazi, their own self-designation. On shifting Laz and Lazi identities and stereotypes, see Meeker (1971), Benninghaus (1989), Bellér-Hann (1995) and Hann (1997).

2 On the development of the tea economy, see Hann 1990.

3 The Hemş'inli are a heterogenous group of Armenian origin who traditionally inhabited more upland villages of the Kaçkar mountains, while the villages situated closer to the coast were mainly occupied by the Lazi.

4 For a detailed description of these baskets see Feurstein (1983:60) and Rize'de el sanatlar 1991:6–7, 22–24.

5 Rize'de el sanatlar (1991:22).

6 Fieldwork among the Lazi was carried out in Turkish as I have no

competence in Lazuri; but whenever possible, informants were asked to name and write down the Lazuri equivalent of a term or a sentence. This was often difficult, because knowledge of Lazuri is uneven and varies according to village, age, gender and education, and because it is not a written language. Literate informants are literate only in Turkish. For one man's extraordinary attempt to give the Lazi a script, see Feurstein (1984).

7 My rendering of Turkish utterances follows local pronunciation rather than standard Turkish.

8 This is a quotation from my field diary in 1992. Since that time this woman has been married to a Lazi man in a nearby village.

9 As is clear from informants' understanding, the metaphor is understood as expressing both similarity (in its procreational sense) and an interaction (in its productive sense) between the objects involved. Cf. Searle's criticism of the two schools of metaphor theory (1979:99).

10 The Black Sea joke or *Karadenizli fikra* is a well-known genre of local oral tradition.

11 Golden jewellery nowadays is obligatorily given to the bride by the groom's family and it is customarily kept by the woman upon divorce regardless of which party was considered to be at fault and the length of the marriage. The gold is said to be the price paid to the woman for her virginity.

12 Decisions about the children after divorce are usually made by courts.

13 A missing link in Delaney's argument. It is possible that this line of argument could also be used when a girl was born instead of a much-wanted boy. This, however, remains speculation since informants were unable to confirm this.

14 The correct spelling of the word derived from an Arabic stem and a Persian prefix in Turkish is *namahrem*. The concept will also be mentioned in the second part of this paper since it is also well known in Uighur. The correct transliteration of the Uighur form would be *namähräm*. To avoid alternative forms in the same paper I have chosen the form *namahram* throughout which more closely follows the Arabic-Persian usage.

15 My present definition of the concept does not cover all aspects of its usage and understanding in the local context. An excellent elaboration on the concept, albeit within the Shiite context, is that of Khatib-Chahidi (1981).

16 On cousin marriages in Turkey see, for example, Stirling and Incirlioğlu (1996).

17 Cf. Delaney (1991:115). When questioned about the division of labour, most Lazi men maintain that their women work harder than they do themselves. Many say they want to see this changed, but few actually take action in this direction. As if in self-defence, many add that women perform these tasks willingly, without being forced to do so (Turkish: *zorlama yok*). Others point out that in former times women had to use baskets because animals could not be used on the dangerously steep, narrow paths. Women usually give a similar account. They do not describe men as lazy: although most men do

not participate in carrying loads, they work as lorry drivers, workers in local tea factories or have a business in town, and husbands who are away as migrant workers are mostly perceived as hard workers.

18 For a general introduction to the Uighurs see, for example, Lattimore (1950) and Benson (1993a).

19 Fieldwork was carried out in the oasis of Kucha, mainly in the town through open-ended, informal interviews, and in two villages near Kashgar in the form of officially supervised, formal interviews. All interviews were conducted in Uighur – most informants had very little or no knowledge of Chinese. Asking Uighurs about procreation metaphors in China is complicated by the fact that any topic which could possibly be related to sexuality has been highly politicized by the Chinese authorities since the so-called Chinese Salman Rushdie affair in 1989 (Gladney 1991:293, 1992). Since I was always accompanied by a male Chinese academic, and occasionally by local cadres as well, the shyness of Muslim women was particularly hard to overcome. Ideas and practices surrounding birth and birth control are also sensitive issues because of the implementation of the government's family planning policies, now extended to the minorities as well as the Han Chinese.

20 This is particularly remarkable in this case since in his discussion of other topics the same author often resorts to this device.

21 Of the numerous expressions for becoming pregnant, the most commonly used among peasants are: *qosaqta qal* ('it remains in the stomach/belly', referring to the seed) and *qosaq kötär* (= 'to lift the stomach/belly'). The first makes implicit reference to the seed, the second focuses on the female body only.

22 Although it appears to have been more common among the poor. Cf. Benson 1993b; Mackerras 1995:72–3.

23 The recent economic reforms which are presently being implemented in the People's Republic of China give *de facto* ownership of small plots of land to Uighur farmers without legal entitlement. Reviving pre-1949 traditions, many farmers have started to pass on land to their offspring as part of their patronym. However, since fertile land in the oases situated along the fringes of the Taklamakan desert is scarce, the plots in question tend to be very small, a factor which further fosters and reinforces gender asymmetry in matters of inheritance. On the economic conditions of Uighur peasants in the reform era, see Bellér-Hann (1997).

24 It is worth noting that Jarring's information was collected in the late 1920s, while Tenishev's data were collected in 1956. Food as sexual symbol is also used elsewhere: according to an indigenous description from the end of the nineteenth century, if a newly married bride turned out not to be a virgin on her wedding night, a flat bread with a whole in its middle was prepared and shown to the bride's parents (Katanov and Menges [1993]1976:1206–7).

25 This is also closely connected to assumptions about the influence of food on the human body.

26 If the woman is more passionate at the time when the baby is

conceived, she will have a girl; if her husband, a boy will be conceived.

27 Although nowadays even some village women have heard of fertility treatments available in far-away Ürümçi, this remains beyond the reach of all but a few. The locally available family planning organizations aim at reducing family size, and therefore preventing and interrupting pregnancies.

28 The value placed on virginity is shown in the fact that the dowry required for a virgin is higher than that asked at subsequent marriages. However, in cases of divorce the amount of movable property/goods a woman can take from her husband's house has nothing to do with her virgin state before her marriage: it is measured in terms of the length of her marriage, which is taken as an indicator of how much work she has put into the household. If the divorce takes place shortly after the wedding she is likely to get nothing because she has not rendered enough services to her husband's family.

29 The breaking of pollution taboos by the woman can also have negative effects. Such taboos also apply to sexual intercourse and if a feeding mother fails to take a full ablution following intercourse and feeds her baby in a polluted state her baby is likely to become sick and even die.

30 For an indigenous description of this, see Jarring (1992:29–32).

31 This is the prevalent view in the Kashgar area, but there is considerable regional variation: women in the Aksu and Kucha oases are said to have much more freedom to engage in money-earning activities.

32 In addition to ploughing, the hoe is also important in the digging of irrigation canals, a male job, which is of primary importance in the Uighurs' oasis agriculture.

CHAPTER 7

PROCREATION IN ISLAM

A READING FROM EGYPT OF PEOPLE AND TEXTS

HANIA M. SHOLKAMY

INTRODUCTION

This paper is about the relationship between Islam, its interpretation, and gender. I shall address this relationship with particular reference to Egypt.

In examining issues pertaining to gender and its construction, the main focus is on theories of procreation in the context of Islamic thought. Renewed interest in procreation theory and Islam has been driven by Carol Delaney's book *The Seed and the Soil: Gender and Cosmology in Turkish Village Society* (1991). In this ethnography of a Turkish village Delaney relates local beliefs about procreation to gender relations in rural Turkey, the construction of the Turkish state, and the foundations of the monotheistic religion of Islam. Delaney herself is a feminist anthropologist trained in religious thought.[1] Her work is important because her interpretations have been adopted by other researchers and re-applied to other Muslim societies (see Inhorn 1994).

By casting her analytical net far and wide, Delaney has attempted to create another all-encompassing metonymic theory to explain gender in Islam (Appadurai 1988; Abu-Lughod 1993). This theory argues that monogenesis and monotheism are one and the same. The creative and authoritative relationship between God and Man is in some ways echoed by the male human's creativity as provider of semen, and his dominion over his wife. As God is to humans, so husband is to wife.

I am sceptical about how far the metaphors of monogenetic

creativity can explain the complex, often conflicting and diverse beliefs of millions of Muslims. I also reject the immediacy of the link between supposed procreation theory and gender relations. And lastly I question the viability of Delaney's methodological project, which infers from the local to the general, to the Turkish, to the Arabic, to the villager, and to God and back.

In my paper I shall try to justify my reservations and answer some of my own questions. I shall refer to theories of procreation and gender construction in a village in Upper Egypt which was the setting for my doctoral research. In this illustrative section I shall try to relate beliefs on procreation to the centrality of children as prescribed by social and political village life and by the Islamic intellectual heritage of this village. I shall then discuss issues of procreation and the tenets of Islam as they exist in religious and other texts. Following these two sections, I shall present some questions concerning procreation and the construction of gender in an Islamic context, pointing to the relevance of sexuality and roles of motherhood and fatherhood as significant indicators to the understanding of Islam, gender, and the relationships between men, women and children.

PROCREATION THEORIES IN AN EGYPTIAN VILLAGE

Khadra swore that she had a big argument with el-Ghazaly last night. He got angry with her and swore that come the feast he would take another wife. She is his third wife and he is her second husband. As Khadra complained, Aziza replied '*el-mara Laha iyeh gheir awlad-ha?*' (what does a woman have but her children?!)[2].

Men and women in Upper Egypt value their fertility and their progeny. Fertility is not a value in itself, neither is the ability to conceive or cause conception. What matters is the successful completion of conception and the aquisition of the social roles of parenthood.

In the village of Rihan where I did my fieldwork (1991–3) fertility and childbearing presented themselves as the most significant faculties that women and men possess. Rihan is a small village (population 1,200) in the governorate of Assiut. The inhabitants are all Muslim except for a few scattered farmers who are Copts and live on the outskirts of the village, in the proximity of the nearby Coptic church, saint's shrine and cemetery. For all villagers, the ability to conceive and receive live healthy children is an incomparable blessing for both men and women.

> Of course children are a blessing. What would life be like without them? Many a time women have almost lost their lives, lost their minds, even almost lost their religion just to see the fingernail of a child. This is why God created us and it is he that creates children. Here we say, 'The father connects progeny and the mother is a vessel that is emptied' [*Al-ab ye'sib wa Al-om ma'oun we faragh*]. It is a poor woman indeed who does not bear children but women must never lose hope in the ability and will of God. (Ni'mat, 37-year-old mother of nine children).

In Rihan, the child defines gender roles, kinship, power, and indeed the quality of adult existence. To discuss theories of procreation, one must understand the centrality of children to the village and its people. Intercourse and conception are separated from fatherhood and motherhood by a long line of events, responsibilities and risks. By and large, women play a bigger role, and thus bear more responsibility, in the process of delivering a living child. But because children are the issue and due to the historical prevalence of failed pregnancies and neo-natal mortality, men and women in Rihan view the procreative act as one stage of a long process by which children are sought. As one mother who has only six children surviving from twenty-three pregnancies said, 'What does it matter if it is a boy or not, if it is dead!'

My friend Ni'mat explained that the function of the man is to act as a connecting nerve, *ye'sib*. The word *'asab* means nerve in Arabic. According to her the man's function is to connect the nerve which connects the patriliny. The role of the man, then, is to connect and by so doing he establishes the roles and rights of the mother and of his own kin. The same word *ye'sib* is also used in the context of Islamic inheritance laws. According to the law a male son connects (again, the verb *ye'sib*) which means he ensures that his father's estate passes on to himself, his mother and his female siblings and is not shared by male uncles and cousins. Although Ni'mat bestows on women the status of passive vessels, she is not saying that men are life-givers. By passing on sperm to the woman, through his water, the man connects the patriline through the woman. Ni'mat is describing connectivity and kinship roles, not agency and procreative powers. Because kinship is organized according to principles of the patriline, the mother by herself cannot connect a child to an ancestral line.

While men in *Rihan* are thought to have a superior status to that of women they are not deemed to have a greater power of procreation, merely a greater *interest* in having particularly male progeny. Women nurture the foetus that is destined to be part of another lineage. However, with the popularity of endogamous marriages, particularly father's brother's daughter unions, the woman is in many cases delivering her child to her own patriline.

The political importance of children makes fertility an elevated and essential value. The passionate pursuit of parenthood in *Rihan* is only tempered by a deep belief in God and the many ways in which God challenges his believers. So if a woman falls victim to infertility or to the inability to bear healthy children she can find some solace in her community. Many will argue on her behalf that it is the will of God, which human beings should not challenge. However men do seek other women if their wives are infertile. This is explained as being a 'dearth in faith' (*Qilit Iman*) but this harsh pronouncement is abated and complemented with 'But what can a man do, does he not need children? Maybe he will be lucky with another woman'; and other expressions of understanding and empathy. But when a man has many sons and takes on another woman just to have more this is referred to as 'greed' (*tama'*).

While at one level villagers joke about sex and sexuality, procreation is strictly the work and gift of God. This is made clear in discussions of contraception. A story is told of a woman, as always in a nearby village, who took the contraceptive pill. Her husband consented and said, 'I do not want to make any more!' The story goes that she became pregnant and a deformed baby was born. On one of its hands was written: 'I have created, now you complete the job!' (*Ana khalakt we inte kamil*) and in the other hand the baby clutched a pill. This proved that God has no tolerance for the arrogance of those who think that they make their children or for the stupidity of others who think that they can prevent his will.

Because fertility is viewed as the ability to bear live children and not the ability to conceive, pregnancy is not celebrated in itself. When a new bride becomes pregnant the issue is not publicized. Mayza, for example, became pregnant three months after her wedding. She was 18-years-old. Among the women I knew, I alone considered her pregnancy an event.[3]

Her in-laws and relatives treated it as a matter of course. When she complained of morning sickness and pains she was usually told to shut up by any female relatives who happened to be around. If she did not, she would hear a profusion of comments to the effect that she 'is not the first or the last to bear a child', 'first babies are always difficult but that never stopped anyone having them', 'pregnancy is not a cause for complaint', 'did you think that you just lie down next to him [her husband] and that's all there is to it?' and many other formulations of similar meanings.

Once pregnant, the activities of women affect the formation of the foetus. *El-Waham* or cravings must be dealt with whatever the cost. The popular belief is that women suffer from *Waham* and so crave foodstuffs; if they do not get them, the baby will have an imprint of this unsatisfied craving. Amongst the Cairo elite, women crave marrons glacés or rare fruits which the husband dutifully gets. In *Rihan*, women generally crave salty things which are easily obtainable. Husbands acquire the craved foodstuff to satisfy the wife, protect the baby from birthmarks and to prove their love, devotion and tolerance. Mayza craved salted fish which was difficult to get at that time of year but her husband, Hamed, did get her some from Cairo. In the case of women who have delivered many times before, craving is less of an issue and the more children they have, the less concerned husbands are about their cravings. Some women crave mud, clay or gypsum. All three are important sources of iron, minerals and calcium. One woman told me, 'Last time when I was pregnant with 'Amr I crunched my way through nearly a whole clay water pot.'

During pregnancy a mother looks at a picture so that the baby comes out resembling that picture. When Mayza entered her fourth month, posters of female Egyptian movie stars suddenly appeared on the house walls. 'If it is a girl I want her to be beautiful like them so I look at the pictures all day,' she explained. Her mother-in-law said that it was all nonsense and that the foetus was already formed by the will of God from her and her husband. But there is a belief that *el-'irk ymed li-sabe' gid* (the blood vessel connects back to the seventh ancestor) so this baby might resemble any one of his male or female kin. On another occasion, Mayza's mother-in-law scolded her, saying, 'Instead of looking in the mirror, look at his father'. Mayza had been engaged in peering at herself at the mirror so that the baby would resemble her. These anecdotes underline beliefs in the mother's role in forming the foetus.

If a woman has a history of miscarriage or if she has had newborns die frequently, pregnancy is accompanied by apprehension. In this case women pursue several courses of therapy including begging from people so that God gives her or 'begs unto her' (*ye-shahat-oh la-ha rabina*) a child. Women also make amulets which they carry in their clothes or sew into a pillow so that the newborn infant may live. The well-being of the baby is the responsibility of the mother. It is she who needs to beg the intercession of spirits and of God so as to come to full-term pregnancy. So whereas the life of the foetus is bestowed by God, its protection from premature death is thought to be in the hands of the mother.

THE PREFERENCE FOR A SON

> Women here have no religion. When it is a boy they say 'she got a boy' but when it is a girl they say 'God sent a girl'. It is God who sends both but they try to take the credit for getting a son. (Om Khattab, the local midwife)

Throughout Upper Egypt there is a strong preference for male children and at the moment of delivery the greatest concern is the sex of the baby. The sex of the child is, at one deep level of faith, believed to be the will of God. One man who has sons said, 'There is a prophetic tradition that says if a man has four daughters he goes straight to heaven.' This is explained as a way by which Islam rewards those who have been deprived of the right and honour of having sons to carry their names. But also it is compensation for the great difficulties involved in bringing up girls and guarding their honour and well-being.

Hashem, my host in the village, explained to me the importance of sons. 'You know if I had no sons, my name and reputation would perish from this earth when I am gone. I would have to rely on my brothers' sons to remember me and people would only remember me by them.' This concern for being remembered is central to the intellectual and emotional deliberations of men in Rihan.[4] Girls do not pass on the father's name. They also owe their allegiance and work to the family of their husbands. There is a popular saying that girls leave behind an empty space (*el-banat marbet-hon khaly*). This refers to the disappearance of girls from their homestead once they are married. When a woman enters another home due to marriage, her ties with her own family cease to involve obligation, and will be purely emotional for the rest of her life, unless she separates from her husband.

Male children are also important for women. Motherhood bestows them with an immediate status. Women acquire the title of 'Om' (mother) followed by the name of the first baby. This title is carried with pride. Now she is a real Om. Until giving birth a married woman may be called Om because of her own father. So for example I was called Om Mohammed because Mohammed is my father's name and partially in anticipation of the boy that I may have. Women who keep trying to have a child but fail are called Om el-Ghayeb which means 'mother of the absent one' (Inhorn 1994).

The name Om so-and-so is the first thing that a new mother hears as the woman who delivers her usually says, 'Thank God for your safety, you have given birth to a boy Om so and so' (*hamd lil Allah ala el salama gibty wald ya Om . . .*). The name of the first boy is never a mystery. It is the name of the husband's father, unless there are other grandchildren bearing that name, in which case the woman may be called 'mother of the new-born' (Om el-mawloud). Modern couples such as Mayza and Hamed may have already picked a name before she delivers.

If the first-born is a girl the mother is also called Om followed by the girl's name. This of course does not have the same ring to it and is often done just to make the mother feel better about herself and to celebrate her motherhood regardless of the gender of the baby.

The question of who is responsible for the generation of a male child has answers in the realm of folklore and custom. 'They say on television and in the clinics that it is the man who decided if the baby is a boy or a girl,' said Mayza. This favourite topic of conversation inspires many lines of thought. Typically, the man feels free to shun the responsibility of the sex of the child and blames it on his wife, whom he may desert if she gives birth to daughters only. But women are not averse to this logic since many a bride is married off on the basis that 'her folk beget sons'. This point of marriageability is seductive to men. Accordingly the responsibility of the sex of the child is borne by either man or woman according to the success or failure of their union.

Hashem's brother has nine sons. 'It is my seed, I begot them from three different women,' he said. On the other hand when their elder brother, who was dying of cancer, and had as yet no sons, wanted to get married, the family nominated a middle-aged widow who had given her previous husband six healthy sons. She did not want to marry but she was talked into it.

The birth of a girl however is never lamented. First for religious reasons: 'It is God who sends, not we who create. Can anyone create a finger nail?!' is a typical retort. But in the case of women who are still young, older mothers will say cheerfully that her *Nassib* (lot or share but more accurately fate/destiny) remains. 'As long as there is one boy to keep the house open, then whatever God sends is a blessing.' One grandmother said as she fondled her new-born granddaughter (who was 30 days old), 'You! You will enliven a home and bear boys,' and laughed at such a distant but wonderful prospect.

With the birth of a boy, a mother acquires status. With the birth of a girl, she is assured of her fertility and she can go on trying for a son. And it is always made clear that girls are 'a gift from God' (*'atiyet rabina*) and are cherished as much as boys are.

'Aziza's is a case in point. She is a young woman in her mid-twenties. She is married to Ragab who is an occasional labourer in Libya. She lives with his mother, older unmarried sister, younger marriageable sister and his brother who is 14 years old. She has two daughters of her own aged 5 years and 4 years. In February 1992 she had another girl. The baby was delivered by 'Aziza's mother and aunt. Her grandmother from her father's side decided to call her Karima after her own eldest daughter. The father was absent abroad and when they found it to be a girl they felt no urgency to wire him with the news.

When I went to see 'Aziza, a few hours after her dawn delivery, she was lying on some mats on the floor covered with a tattered quilt. Around her were two of her sisters, her sister-in-law and mother-in-law, her aunt and her cousin and neighbour. Her daughters were being chased by their aunt who wanted to bathe them. 'Be gentle and let them wear what they want,' 'Aziza shouted out to her sister-in-law. Then she explained to me that they had both been there when she delivered and that they had become very nervous and the youngest was frightened. As she said this, Sawsan, her eldest daughter, crouched and began to imitate her mother giving birth while the younger girl, Racha, made as if she was receiving the child. Their mother told me that she had overheard them saying, 'Now our mother will take off her trousers and get a baby.' Their grandmother explained their nervousness by saying, 'Poor girls, they sat up crying all night because they wanted a brother.'

I had anticipated 'Aziza's worry because her new-born was not a boy. Her mother-in-law told me that she is young and that there is still hope for her to bear Ibrahim[5]. She added that 'Aziza was very tired and quiet because girls are always more difficult to deliver than boys. They are heavier, gestate for a longer period of time, and take time to deliver. This is an observation and a belief that is commonly held in the village. Mothers say, 'I had an easy delivery although it was a girl,' as Ni'mat told me. she had her lates. 'Aziza was also suffering from post-partum pains known in Upper Egypt as *Om el-Khawalef* which means 'mother of those who deliver'. They had sent for some painkillers which were called the *Om el-Khawalef* pill. Actually it was an anti spasmodic. *Om el-Khawalef* has nothing to do with the gender of the child. It is something which most women get and which is made more severe if post-partum blood is delayed. 'Aziza's mother however had an explanation which was supported by three of the women present and rejected by two. She said, 'Perhaps when 'Aziza was sitting on the bricks [*el-qawalib*] and was told that it was a girl, she held in her blood out of disappointment!'

'Aziza was disappointed but thankful that it was over. She was also proud of her beautiful baby daughter, whom she began to feed the next day. 'Ragab won't throw me out,' she joked several months after her delivery. 'He is not exactly a millionaire to need an heir.' Aside her mother told me that Ragab and 'Aziza are cousins, so he will not harm her. If anything, it is 'Aziza who comes from the larger and richer part of the family. The fact is that despite this being her third daughter, there was only a sense of disappointment, not of panic.

But for some women, having no sons also means having no property, no home, no family and no source of income. El-Ziniyeh has only daughters. She lives alone in a small mud house. Her daughters are married. One is in the village and the other two are in Arab Matteer. They are all married to cousins. El-Ziniyeh used to work even when her husband was still alive. Her three brothers are perhaps the wealthiest men in the village, largely because they have been working in Saudi Arabia for 20 years and operate a thriving business in visa procurement for others. Because of this elevated status, they have stopped their eldest sister, el-Ziniyeh, from working. She used to sell eggs in the market and run errands, sell and shop for other women. Her brothers have ordered her to be discreet about her activities.

El-Ziniyeh was pointed out to me as one of the poorest women in the village and one who leads a wretched life *(ghalbana)*.

> What can daughters do for me? When I visit, they get worried that I will upset their mothers-in-law. As for my brothers, well, brothers give their goodness *[kheir]* to their wives and a bit of meat and their anger [*ghadab*] to their sisters. If I had a son, wouldn't his knock on my door and his entrance be like an angel stepping through the gates of heaven?!

As she spoke, Karima told her, 'Don't make it worse for yourself, don't lose your religion now.' Women like her really have no source of income except that which they get from their work and the pittance of a pension (in 1994 it was six Egyptian pounds a year, which equals approximately £1.50 sterling) which they receive from the government, known as the Sadat pension. Om Zeinab is in the same situation, only she has one daughter who is married in Arab Matteer and no brothers. There are another three women like them in the northern part of the village. Ni'mat explained that they are the ones who really deserve charity. During harvests, people send them some crops, which they can eat or sell. They also go out to work as day labourers during harvest times. Then they go back to the field and pick up any leftovers (these are known as *Al-sayf* and are particularly lucrative at the cotton harvests).

Such is the lot of widows who have no sons. This is partly why fertility and male children are needed in several different kinds of ways. In their day-to-day life, women without sons feel the pain of their disability. They also pay a clear price. With children, and especially sons, women create families in which they have an elevated status.

Persistently, villagers stressed that it is God who creates, lamented the faithlessness of men who blamed their wives for their inability to bear children or bear boys, empathized with the efforts of these same men in searching for progeny and another wife, and laughed at women who tried to convince their husbands that they, the wives, and not God, had produced sons. For me, the main conclusion from these discussions is people's heightened sense of context and of the politics of reproduction. They stressed that people only begin to think about these things when their reproductive strategies fail, and that true belief in God means acceptance and adjustment but does not deny the human being the right to try to change an umpromising situation.

VARIETIES OF ISLAM IN RIHAN

Rihan is a largely Muslim community which is not cut off from its Islamic intellectual and jural heritage. The village is the site of religious debate and contemplation. The men and women with whom I worked in Rihan have access to three 'kinds' of religious instruction and thought. The most pervasive is the religious thinking and opinion provided by local preachers. Since the village does not have a large mosque regulated by the ministry of *Awqaf*,[6] it does not have an official sheikh educated in Al-Azhar, the official Islamic university. The local preachers are all men who apprenticed as sheikhs and who recite the Quran on demand. They also lead the Friday prayers. The favourite is sheikh Mostafa, a blind man who recites the Quran during funerals and during religious commemorations.

On one such occasion, sheikh Mostafa was invited by Om Ragab for the annual commemoration of her husband's death. He came and sat outside the house to recite the Quran while men came to pay their condolences. In between recitations he was invited in to have his tea with the women inside the house. When 'Aziza came with the tea she put a glass in his hand and said,

'Here is your tea, now preach.' He complied and started to explain matters of religion to the assembled women. He talked about inter-marital relations. Following are some excerpts:

> The duty of the wife is to go to the bed of the husband. Even if she is baking, even if she is baking and he calls her she must go.[7] No matter what she is doing or what he smells like, even if he smells like a corpse she must go to him. If she doesn't he has the right to punish her. I am not talking about the stick. The husband can desert her for up to three months. The prophet himself, the praise of Allah be upon him, once said that a woman who will not leave her baking to go to her husband will burn in a fire worse than that of the oven.

'Aziza, and Kamla her friend were scandalized. 'He can desert her for three months, this is too much,' they said laughing. 'Aziza's mother-in-law commented aside, 'This is enough to make 'Aziza behave.'

The sheikh, like others with a similar background, is considered a member of the family. He is invited inside the home and he preaches a religion that is 'culturally adjusted' to the needs and knowledge of the village. He was undoubtedly placing words in the mouth of the prophet since no such prophetic tradition exists. These sheikhs are usually friendly and talk in a vernacular tongue. They make allowances for folk beliefs without preaching blasphemy. They preach an accommodating philosophy which draws on classical orally transmitted interpretations from the Hanafi school of jurisprudence. For example, sheikh Mostafa does not scold women who do not perform regular prayers since he says, 'Here women always have a legitimate excuse not to pray.' He is referring to menstruation, post-partum blood and the need to purify oneself after intercourse. He commented jokingly, 'Of course all Muslims must pray, but our women would dissolve from all the water they would have to purify themselves in.'

Rihan is a village that has many sons affiliated with Egyptian Islamic fundamentalism. Ni'mat's brother is one of the 'brothers', so are many of his friends and cousins. Their influence in the village has been great. Before being imprisoned, as they all are now, they took over the Friday sermons in the mosques. They outlawed saint's day celebrations and other such festivities. They discouraged people from watching television. They went round the houses telling their female relatives to pray and fast. They imposed the veil on their relatives, advising that girls as young as 7 years old must veil. They campaigned against the women who did not pray, mentioning their names in public and refusing to greet them.

These zealots are staunch followers of the teachings of Ibn Taymiyya which are inspired by the Hanbali school of jurisprudence. They are literalists and fundamentalists. They have many emulators in the village. During one marriage celebration some of these emulators came to greet the groom. When they walked in the tape recorders were switched off and all the dancing and smoking were abandoned. This school of thought has shaped the culture of the village, and its emergence is often referred to as an event in the life of the village and one which set right the beliefs and practices of villagers.

In addition to these schools of thought there is the official Islamic thinking that is taught in schools, preached on the radio and television, and disseminated by officials and professionals such as schoolteachers and doctors during their encounters with villagers. This religious thinking is a politically adjusted Islam that preaches Hanafi principles but espouses conformity, modernity and government support.

These three sources of intellectual thought (local sheikh, fundamentalists and offical modernist Muslims) are very much part of people's day-to-day life. But they are resources that are activated upon demand. When I asked sheikh Mostafa about the right of a man to take on another wife if his own could not beget sons, this was his answer:

> It is the will of God if a man has sons or not. When Om Shihata was losing her babies, I told her that she must make a delicious meal of stuffed pigeons for her husband the minute they come back from the cemetery where they bury their lost ones. Then they should meet, and with the will of God she will get a son. But there is nothing stronger then the will of God but a man has a right to try with another Muslim woman and perhaps God will bless her, this other one with a son.

I put the same question to a friend of one of the radical

Muslim youth of the village. He told me he would ask the sheikh of the mosque which he frequents who is a follower of Ibn Taymiyya and bring me back the reply. The response was that procreation is the undisputed will of God. The prophet himself did not have a son to outlive him. One must accept totally the will of God and it is blasphemy to say it is the man and the woman who are responsible. But no one can deny the absolute right of a man, as it is enshrined in the Quran, to take more than one wife.

On several occasions I spoke to the physicians working in the public clinics that villagers from Rihan use. One physician is a veiled and friendly woman who has worked for almost a decade in the region. I asked her the same question. She replied, 'They are ignorant, they can hardly feed themselves but they want more children and more wives. Let me tell you, our religion is one of acceptance, they think that a child will change their lives ... let me tell you, they are the reason for our sorry state here in Egypt.'

Despite this wealth of religious instruction there is much in village life that is secular. Procreation is Islamicized when it is problematic. There is no denial that God is the creator and procreator. But the minutiae of who is responsible for what are discussed in a secular context unless religious arbitration is sought. It is then that villagers call upon these various resources to justify or rationalize chosen courses of action.

FROM ALLAH TO ATA?!

To return to Delaney: she quotes from the Quran the verse that tells the believer that 'Women are given to you as fields to be sown, so go to them and sow [your seed] as you wish.' She notes that God is speaking to men about women, thus women are excluded and objectified. In this she presents the locus of the relationship between God, man and women (Delaney 1991:30). Her view is that this act of procreation and the language used by the Quran to describe it are culturally constructed and ideological.

She maintains that men pass *can* (life/soul in Turkish) through their seed to the soil that nurtures this seed, which is the woman's womb. Just as God created life single-handedly, so do they generate seed and therefore procreate monogenetically. She carries on this imagery and maps onto it congruent interpretations of intercourse, daily language, menstruation and afterbirth taboos, virginity, veiling, gender relations within marriage, and the construction of Turkish identity, society and the State.

Perhaps one can read Delaney as having written an ethnography of specific Turkish interpretations of Islam and of gender. If indeed daily language, life, sexuality and gender are thus metaphorized with references to man as God and as life-giver and woman as field and nurturer, then procreation is the key to an understanding of rural life and people in Turkey. But Delaney proposes that this metaphorization and symbolism also reflect a wider Islamic reality. She quotes the prominent sheikh el-Ghazaly, citing him as a monogeneticist (Delaney 1991:288). She makes a leap from *Allah* (father in Turkish) to *Ata* (ancsstor), relying on the work of scholars like F. Sabbah (1984), A. Bouhdiba (1985), and others.

El-Ghazaly wrote *Ihya' 'Oloum ed-Deen* (*The Renaissance of Religious Learning*) at the beginning of the twelfth century. The second part of this work is about the *adab* (rules/etiquette) of cohabitation. Part 10 of this volume he devotes to sexual intercourse. There he states:

> The foetus is not created from the man alone but from both partners together either from his water and her water or from his water and her menstrual blood. Some anatomists have said that the embryo is created of menstrual blood. (El-Ghazaly 1990:5)

Undoubtedly, el-Ghazaly believes that Islam holds a duogenetic theory of conception even if in other parts of his opus he does suggest the prominence of the role of the man in procreation. In fact, creation in Islam is God's work. Man and woman are vehicles through which the miracle of creation occurs through the intercession of God (Morsy 1988). Every single incidence of conception is God's and not that of the man or the woman. The Quran does tell men to 'sow their fields' as Delaney put it but this *Aya* (miracle/verse) does not mention any creative or procreative act in connection with sowing the field. The sense of the *Aya* relates to procreation and to intercourse. The Quran is specific in its depiction of the creation and development of the human foetus. According to the *Igma'* (consensus) of scholars the stages of creation and gestation are: a chain of mud, then a *nitfa* (morsel), *Alaqa* (clot of blood), *Madgha* (embryo), bones, flesh, another being. Each stage takes 40 days and 40 nights during which the embryo is enclosed in the mother's womb. When the embryo is a *Madgha* God announces four words which will specify: its future wealth, the hour of its death, the work it will do, and whether it is to be happy or sad. Then, and only then, God grants the embryo the miracle of life (Al-Azhar 1992:7).

This religious view of gestation and creation is not merely symbolic or allegorical; it is of extreme juridical and temporal significance. For example, the Hanafi school allows for justified abortion before the passage of 120 days of gestation since the foetus is as yet not a living soul. Schools differ in what they accept as justifications for abortion. The Hanafi school accepts the mother's fear of not being able to take care of older children as an excuse for abortion. Other schools demand that no excuse less than jeopardy to the mother's health is acceptable. The Zaidi school gives women the absolute right to make this decision. The Hanafi school reiterates its belief that the embryo does not count as a living soul before 120 days by making the mother exempt from paying any kind of compensation for the taking of the life of the foetus, since it does not yet have the breath of life from God.

Islam does not deny the positive role played by men and women in the genetic composition of a child. In *Aya* 14 of *Surat el-Molk* it says 'choose well for your progeny', advising Muslims to be careful in their choice of marriage partners. This is not only an indication of the nurturing role of the mother but also of her genetic role. Unlike accepted stereotypes and actual practices the prophet and his followers discouraged endogamy because it resulted in weak and sickly offspring.

Another indication of the relevance of both partners to procreation is the *Igma'* that exists concerning contraception. All schools agree that it must be by mutual consent and there are countless texts which admonish men not to practise coitus interruptus without the consent of their wives. The debate that exists in ancient texts concerns the right of a man to withhold his seed from slaves. Some schools give men this unilateral right during intercourse with slaves but not with their 'free' wives (Al-Azhar 1992:31).

The Quran is explicit in denying man the ability to give life. *Ayat* 57–9 of *Surat el-Waqi'a* says, 'We have created you if you would believe have you seen what you desire Did you create or are we the creators?' There is a prophetic tradition (Hadith) which states: 'The water that comes out of you if gushed onto a rock, God could create a son from it'. While this tradition could be taken to mean that a woman can be replaced by a rock, it also withdraws from semen the procreative capacity, making this power that of God alone.

Even when referring to the act of agriculture itself, the text of the Quran is as explicit about the will of God being the only power which can engender plants, not just men and women. In *Ayat* 24–32 of *Surat 'Abas*, the Quran says 'Let the human being look at his food. We poured the water and parted the soil and inseminated it with seeds and grapes and trees and olives and palms and gardens that are full and many fruits for your pleasure and benefit/nourishment.' Whether a human or plant seed, it is still a vehicle of God-given life and in that it is no different from the womb or soil which accepts and nurtures it.

Procreation in Islamic texts and scholarship is not a male act, but it is a sacred one. When men are advised to mention the name of God at the point of intercourse this is not necessary to reaffirm the camaraderie between *Ata* and *Allah*. The name of God is enjoined during any sacred act and, in Islamic thinking, legitimate intercourse which could lead to conception is such an act (Morsy 1988; Delaney 1991; Mernissi 1991; Ali 1996).

The above citations and those used by Delaney are open to many interpretations. But this takes me back to my previous point. The anthropologist would be advised to take into account the legacy of interpretation and the debates that do exist in so far as they are relevant to the site of fieldwork. Analysts also need to retain some order of magnitude when structuring an argument out of cited works. For example, when citing prophetic traditions, we should say whether they are contested *Hadith* or widely accepted ones. This order of legitimacy, integrity and magnitude of Islamic texts is central to Islamic scholarship (Mernissi 1991). Otherwise the relationship between Islam and ethnography will remain an awkward one.

The question that remains unanswered is why the language of procreation is metaphorized in the way that it is. One can offer only a conjectural answer. One alternative is to think in terms of the immobile field which accepts mobile seed. The relationship between the womb and the child to be born is similar to that between fields and their yet-to-be harvested crops. Seeds however are transient and may be ploughed in more than one field. These metaphors of seed and soil may be metaphors of sexual intercourse and of human physiology as well as of procreation.

The interpretation of texts and meaning of the Quran is a discipline in itself. But the Quran is accessible to all, including anthropologists, and its reading is denied to none except women in their temporary state of impurity due to menstruation or after birth. Any Muslim who can read Arabic can and should read the text. Those who cannot read, but understand Arabic, hear its recitation on the radio or on tapes. However there are *adab* (rules/etiquette) of interpretation and citation which need to be kept in mind if one is to draw any meaningful conclusions concerning Islam as based on the practices of Muslims.

THE STUDY OF PROCREATION AND GENDER

In challenging the argument that Islam holds a monogenetic theory of procreation, I am not denying that it is a patriarchal religion which holds a world view that favours men over women. Delaney blames Paternity for the situation of Muslim women (Delaney 1986:495). I would like to argue a more traditional point and relate gender and its construction to patriarchy.

To understand or address the situation of women in Islam one needs to look at the legal aspects of kinship and property which Islam has promoted and not just at its theories of procreation.

Islamic law makes children the property of the patriline. The kinship and property rules which define the situation of children do not rely on a biological explanation nor are they apologetic about their treatment of women. An example from present-day Egypt may serve to illustrate. In Egypt women do not have the right to pass on their nationality to their children. The thousands of poor women who married oil-rich Arab summer tourists who come to Egypt for a good time have brought this issue to the top of the feminist and the political agendas. These women are very often deserted by their husbands and may be left pregnant (IRRRAG 1996). They cannot give their children an Egyptian nationality, and unless they have the father's support to prove paternity they cannot get them passports from the embassy of the country of origin of the father.

Feminists have been debating this point for decades. The position of Islam does not even enter the discussion because Islamic tenets espouse a duogenetic theory of procreation and because the question is not a religious one. The position of the courts of Cairo is that dual citizenship is problematic if the 'primary' citizenship, that which is passed on by the father, is not an Egyptian one. The debate centres around security and national allegiance and not around seed and soil.

In the case of these abandoned women and their children, the facts of procreation are irrelevant. The political reality is the nature of the power relationships between Egypt and rich Arab neighbours. Egyptian embassies in these countries dare not chase the usually happily married father nor will they support the claims of these women and their advocates. Patriarchy and a morality which blames these women for marrying strangers are at the root of this persistent problem. The facts or beliefs concerning procreation have no bearing on rules of kinship or on the legal and jural rights of men and women. Semen and egg are in themselves not sanctified.

CONCLUSION

I have tried to make a number of ethnographic and methodological contributions to an understanding of the relationship between procreation theories and Islam. From a methodological point of view, I have tried to raise the issue of texts and intellectual context in relation to ethnographic research in societies where the majority are not effectively literate. To comment on the beliefs and practices of societies, one needs to take into account the intellectual heritages and discursive traditions, and to engage with them rather than ignore them in favour of pure observation.

As far as Islam is concerned, I contest the monogenetic thesis argued by Delaney (1991) and Inhorn (1994), and show that there is enough in terms of written text and judgement to render the Islamic theory of procreation, at the human biology level, a duogenetic one; actually it is *theo-genetic*, a theory in which God is the sole source of creation. This does not mean that the patriarchy of Islam is less real. The work of Mernissi (1991) and Ahmed (1992) attempted to understand the male bias in Islam by reference to its theological, juridical and interpreted history. In this quest lies the key to the perceived misogyny of some Islamic interpretations.

Theories of procreative biology reflect, rather than determine, wider political ideologies. To understand procreation, we must consider property law, sexuality and gender roles. My argument is that gender defines the physical and biological relationship between men and women. The obligations and privileges of parenthood are one key determinant of gender roles. Any male bias that exists in Egyptian societies has political and economic, and not just biological, justifications.

The ethnographic data presented show the centrality of children as social beings to the lives of men and women. They reveal fatherhood and motherhood as roles of consequence to society. The ethnography also shows that this remote village has an intellectual and jural Islamic heritage but, despite this, still retains an element of secularity that is often ignored by analysts working amongst Muslims. This view of the village as a site of confluence of intellectual and religious thought is a necessary context for understanding the village itself, and for understanding more profoundly the issues raised by Delaney.

NOTES

1 Delaney says in her 1991 book that she trained at the Harvard School of Divinity.

2 The word *awlad* comes from the root *walad* which means boy. But the word for delivery is *wilada*. Generally, *awlad* is used to mean children but in rural Egypt it usually implies male children only. A classic misunderstanding occurs when urbanites ask women, 'How many *awlad* do you have?', meaning children, and she replies 'One', meaning that she has one son, although she may have five daughters as well.

3 Moreover, the mere thought of pre-natal care was met with consensus as to *my* eccentricities. It is basically not done. Specialists, whether they are local or government health professionals, can confirm pregnancy but have no role to play except in termination of pregnancy, whether by abortion, miscarriage or delivery.

4 This village is illustrative of the culture of Upper Egypt. It is in no way unique or spectacular.

5 Ibrahim is the name of 'Aziza's father-in-law who died three years before this paper was published.

6 This is the ministry which handles religious properties and endowments.

7 A woman can only leave her baking in the event of an emergency since the dough would spoil and the fire would go out if both are left unattended. This is gross waste and is something that is never done.

The translation of the meaning of verse from the Quran is the author's own.

CHAPTER 8

THE LIGHT OF LIFE

REPRESENTATIONS OF PROCREATION, DIVINITY AND PROPERTY IN CARNIA AND ANATOLIA

PATRICK HEADY

This paper is primarily about Carnia, a mountainous area in the extreme northeast of Italy, where I did fieldwork between 1989 and 1991. In Carnia, as in many other parts of southern Europe, people associate generative processes in both humans and plants with various forms of light (Pina-Cabral; 1986; Verdier 1990; du Boulay 1991). This idea, which is sometimes taken literally and at others evoked figuratively, often seems to be elaborated for its own sake; but it also provides a way of expressing relationships between different kinds of biological and spiritual energy, and between different orders of living being. This paper has two aims: to explore the range of imagery in which light is involved, and to analyse the system of relationships – between procreation, social categories, divinity and property – which the imagery helps to express.

I will use the results to comment on two recent accounts of the social significance of procreative images and ideas. Bloch and Parry (1982) argue that the imagery often contrasts two distinct kinds of fertility: firstly, the disorderly and corruptible forces of natural fertility, associated particularly with women; and secondly, an image of pure incorruptible divine fertility which can only be attained through the acceptance of death. The imagery of divine fertility is controlled by senior men, and reinforces their power. Another author who has made strong claims about the strength and directness of the connection between social structure and the imagery of generative power is Delaney (1986,1991). She traces systematic connections between three spheres of culture and social organization: firstly, monotheistic religion which ultimately traces all creativity to a single divine source; secondly, a doctrine of procreation in which only one of the two sexual roles – that of the man – is seen as legitimate; and thirdly, agriculture and the social implications of the inseminating role of male agriculturalists.

In this paper I will make frequent reference both to Delaney's arguments and to her findings, which were based on fieldwork in a village in Anatolia. Though Anatolian society and Carnian society differ in important ways, they have enough in common for comparisons to be worth making. Both contain small nucleated villages. Until the 1960s Carnians depended for much of their subsistence on a combination of agriculture and livestock raising, in which each patrilocal three-generation family was a separate agricultural unit, but in which the village as a whole cooperated in the management of collective property or cooperative enterprises. Much the same set-up was still in operation in Anatolia at the time (around 1980) when Delaney did her fieldwork. On the other hand the religious context was very different. Although Delaney herself argues that Christianity and Islam understand procreation in much the same way, I will try to show that the two religious ideologies interact with ideas about procreation itself in ways that have different spiritual and social implications.

LIGHT AND THE POWERS OF PHYSICAL GENERATION

In Carnia life force can take the form of sunlight, moonlight or sparks of fire. The next few paragraphs outline some of the main features of this scheme. Among the points which emerge, and which will be important for later parts of the paper, are the parallels between people and plants, the association of some generative processes with disorder, and the difference between the ways men and women relate to the forces involved.

People say comparatively little about the generative power of the sun. This is not because its power is discounted, either practically or symbolically. Perhaps the sun's power is too obvious to need discussion; or perhaps the reason is that its social implications, which will emerge later, are relatively uncontroversial. But one thing that does emerge from what people say is the parallel between human impulses and the sun's effect on plants. This is expressed in a charming phrase that is used of plants at the time their leaves are growing and buds are appearing in the spring. They are said to be in *amôr*[1] – that is, in love.

A wide range of biological processes are thought to be affected by the phases of the moon. The waxing moon is associated with biological vigour. Wine bottled when the moon is growing will be fizzy, while wine bottled when the moon is waning will be flat. Sap is thought to rise when the moon is waxing, which means that fruit and vegetables should not be picked at that time – since being full of life they will not come away easily from the plant and afterwards may sprout shoots. Other examples of the moon's influence seem to embody a different principle – a contrast between things which grow upwards and things which grow downwards. Thus corn should be planted when the moon is waxing because it grows upwards, but potatoes should be planted when the moon is waning because they grow under the soil. Beans appear to be an exception to this because they should be planted when the moon is waning, but the reason for this conforms to the general principle. If they were planted when the moon was waxing all their vitality would go into flowering; planting them when the moon is waning ensures that the growth goes into the downward-hanging pods.

The elderly woman who gave me the most complete account of lunar influences insisted that all the moon's influence followed a single principle. At the time I was puzzled by how this applied in the case of plants, since half the examples seemed to relate to growth and vigour as such, while the other half seemed to refer to the direction of the growth. However, these contrasts could be reduced to a single dimension if what I previously glossed as 'biological vigour' was thought of instead as 'outward movement'. In that case there would be a single contrast between upward-and-outward movement, and downward-and-inward movement.

There certainly are clear parallels between the moon's influence on plants and its impact on people and pigs. Hair and beards grow faster when the moon is waxing. If a pig is butchered during the waxing moon its vital forces will be too strong and the meat will quickly go bad. In the days before washing machines sheets were washed when the moon was waning. This fact, which I was told with embarrassed laughs, was because the dirt – presumably including stains from bodily fluids – was more vigorous when the moon was waxing, and so harder to wash out.

The moon is also thought to influence human reproduction.

There is a belief that babies tend to be born at a particular time – or perhaps particular times – in the lunar cycle. Hospital nurses are said to know this from observation. The elderly woman I mentioned before said that conceptions that occurred when the moon was waxing were more likely to produce boys, while girls were more likely to be conceived when the moon was waning – which suggests that births would follow the same pattern. However other informants appeared unsure about exactly how lunar phases relate to the pattern of births, and it is possible that there are alternative theories.

Although no one said directly that the moon influences women's cycles, there is clearly an association of ideas since people would go on from the topic of lunar influence to talk about the damage that menstruating women can do. They are believed to cause metal to tarnish and plants to wither. They must also not be allowed near pork butchery or sausage-making since they will cause the meat to go bad. (Pigs' own sexual biology is thought to have analogous effects on the quality of their meat. Sows are not slaughtered when they are on heat because their meat would rot – just as it would if they were slaughtered when the moon was waxing.)

A possible connection between fire and vital energy emerges from stories about a set of wood-dwelling beings – the *macarots*.[2] Almost no one now believes in *macarots*, but people still know what they were supposed to be like. They were little men who were capable of transforming themselves, particularly by suddenly growing to a huge size, and were tricksters. They lived in the woods and used to hammer on tree-trunks with wooden sticks. Two accounts seem to link *macarots* to fire and sexuality. Gortani ([1898]1981:147) recounts a tale collected in the nineteenth century. Some girls were resting in the evening after cutting the grass for hay. From the other side of the valley they heard some beautiful music. After a while the music stopped, there was a burst of laughter, and they saw a *macarot* in the form of fire shooting down the hillside on the other side of the valley like a rocket. The other account was produced by an old man whom I asked about *fouc voladi* – literally 'flying fire' – flames which seem to hover in the air though nothing appears to be burning. He said that pine trees need to fertilize each other, which they do by knocking their trunks together. This produces *fouc voladi* which turns into a *macarot*.

If life force can be transmitted by light it can also be absorbed by looking. Youthful fertility is constantly threatened by the envious and old. One of the most powerful ways in which an envious person conveys this power is when she (it usually is she) *ti spia fiss ... cui voi* – 'stares at you fixedly with her eyes'. Some people think that such individuals transmit dark rays from their eyes. Although the power of envy is not only directed against manifestations of fertility, this category does cover many of the potential victims – including flowers, cattle, attractive women and, above all, children. Adult men are much less likely to be victims. Sometimes the harm caused by envy is relatively minor. One elderly woman said that her mother, when a girl, had been complimented by a neighbour on her beautiful hair. When she next combed it she found there were lice in it. Clearly the neighbour had caused this to happen. A young woman told me that when her mother failed to give a neighbour some flowers that she wanted, the flowers concerned were the first to wither. To give a more serious example, another elderly woman attributed the persistent ill-health of her sister's children to the fact that at the time she was sharing a house with an envious aunt (FBW).

The eyes of a dying person can endanger those who are yet to be born. A young woman recounted how her father's final illness occurred when she was pregnant. Although she wanted to visit and care for him, her elderly female relatives were against the idea for fear that contact with the dying man would harm the unborn child. She resisted their pressure and continued to visit her father, but nevertheless when he was on the point of death she allowed herself to be bundled out of the room so that his dying glance should not be fixed on her and so harm the child.

But the eyes' power to appropriate life force is not necessarily malign. In the case of pregnant women it becomes so only if it is frustrated. If a pregnant woman sees something that she wants, it is important to give it to her, since otherwise her child will be born with a birthmark in the shape of the object concerned. It is as though she is absorbing the raw materials for the child from the things she sees around her, and if she is not allowed to appropriate them the child will be born with that bit missing.

PROCREATION AND PATRILINY

Perhaps the best established proposition in the literature on this topic is that the parent who is thought to contribute the most, or the most important, stuff to the child is the one to whose social group the child is assigned. In Anatolia and India the image of the seed and the field is used to suggest that the male contributes the decisive factor (Delaney 1986; Dube 1986). Carnians think – or used to think – of families in patrilineal terms: marriage tends to be patrilocal, the birth of a son used to be wished for in order to carry on the family name, and sons used to inherit the bulk of the family property. So there should be evidence that Carnians believe that the father makes the most important physiological contribution to the formation of the child.

But, if there is such a belief, I did not discover it. This may be because I never asked directly (the issue was not at the top of my research agenda at the time). However, if the belief is present, it is rather curious that the symbolism described above doesn't seem to refer to it either. Nevertheless, the symbolism conforms to patrilineal expectations in other ways, by suggesting that the process of procreation subordinates women to men.

One thing which the symbolism does stress is that women's vital energy is not sufficient by itself for their reproductive role. Women are represented as needing to absorb vital energy, while men are endowed with a surplus – effectively placing women in their debt. The association of the male *macarot* with free-standing light, and the idea that women have a need or power to absorb energy from their environment – in pregnancy and also, in some cases, through the evil eye – are expressions of this idea. The belief that boys are conceived when the moon is waxing and girls when it is waning, associates males with a phase of plentiful and outward-moving energy and females with a phase in which it is moving inwards, implying that this difference between male and female natures is inscribed at the very start of life. There is also some symbolism which associates lustful women with greedy pigs, again suggesting that their basic sexual role is to absorb stuff from men.

Delaney's (1991) analysis of the imagery of the seed and the soil identifies another way in which reproductive imagery might reinforce male power. She notes that the image aligns the male partner in sexual intercourse with the active ploughman and the woman with the passive, dominated, land. This is not a comparison I heard in Carnia – perhaps because I failed to ask the right questions, or perhaps because the plough plays a rather minor role in an environment characterized by steep mountain slopes.

However, Delaney's basic point is consistent with the material I collected. The belief that boys are conceived when the moon is waxing and girls when it is waning is analogous to ideas about planting vegetables and so aligns male sexual fluid with seed and the woman with soil. The *macarots* – which seem to have embodied aspects of male sexuality – were depicted as active, aggressive beings. More directly, the casual assumption – by men at least – that sexual intercourse is an act of domination is illustrated by the use of the word *mona* – slang for vulva – to refer to a man who fails to stand up for himself.

The two ideas of the husband's sexual role – as dominating but also in a sense feeding[3] his wife – seem to be implicd in an anti-marriage song that is popular on festive occasions. In the first verse *he* promises that if she marries him he will give her good food. In the second *she* complains that after marriage all she got to eat was *polenta* and bean pods – not very appetizing – and in the evening she was beaten with a stick. In this mockery of a marriage the husband fails to achieve the correct combination of domination and nourishment which a proper sexual relationship would produce.

DISORDER, GENDER AND DIVINITY

But, although the attribution of more vital force and a dominating sexual role to men is consistent with Delaney's argument, other Carnian ideas diverge from the situation she describes in Anatolia. According to Delaney (1991), Anatolians think that the kind of stuff which men and women bring to procreation is different, and they also contrast the shameful, disorderly sexuality of women with the orderly, clean sexuality of men. The two points are condensed into a single idea. Male sexuality, purified by the rite of circumcision, is identified with the generative power of God, while the female role is seen as earthly and defiling. It is consistent with this that the Islamic heaven is conceived in terms of the eternal continuation of male sexual pleasure.

The comparable ideas in Carnia are arranged into a different pattern. The symbolism of light suggests that, though men and women have different sexual roles and different quantities of vital energy, the kind of energy involved is the same for both sexes. The phase of the moon affects biological processes in both men and women. The sexual emissions of both sexes are symbolically related to forms of light. And the waxing of the moon, which is associated with menstruation in the similarity of its effects on pork butchery, is also associated with virility in the belief that boys are conceived when the moon is waxing. The relation of sexuality to disorder also differs from that in Anatolia. There is an idea that sex is inherently improper. Sexual jokes are referred to as 'dirty' – *sporc* – just as they are in England, but unlike Anatolia the disorderly character of sexuality is not exclusively associated with women. Although menstruation is believed to be dangerously polluting, the disruptive nature of *macarots* suggests that male sexuality is also a source of disorder. The association of men with disorderly sexuality is enacted in the annual *cidulas* ceremony in which the young men suggest suitable (or grotesquely unsuitable) love affairs between the unmarried men and women of the village, to the accompaniment of much sexual innuendo.

Consistently with this, divine purity can be envisaged just as easily in the female form of the Virgin as in the male form of Christ. What matters in this regard is the renunciation of sexuality as such, not the distinction between its male and female forms. The way these sacred figures are depicted or imagined also inverts an aspect of the sexual act which is associated with male dominance, since the Virgin is defined by not having been penetrated by a human male, while Christ is someone whose bodily boundaries have been pierced in the course of his ordeal on the cross.

This difference in the religious evaluation of human sexuality helps to explain a well-known difference between the Islamic and Christian societies situated round the shores of the Mediterranean: namely that in the Islamic societies official religion is largely a male preserve, while in the Christian societies it is women who are religiously observant and men (except for priests) ostentatiously keep their distance from church affairs (Davis 1984). In the case of Carnia and Anatolia, these divergent patterns may be closely linked to two crucial points:

1. that human procreation is experienced in both Anatolia and Carnia as an assertion of male status; and
2. that in Anatolia religion reinforces the symbolic significance of procreation, but in Carnia religion devalues all sexuality.

Taken together these statements imply that Muslim worship reinforces male status and female subordination, while Christian worship does the opposite. If one assumes that people prefer to participate in activities which enhance their sense of self-worth, it is understandable that men are religiously inclined in Islamic societies, and women in Christian ones.

The divergent religious attitudes to sexuality relate in turn to a contrast between the Islamic and Christian attitudes to the central religious concept of sacrifice. In the Islamic view the crucial compact between mankind and God follows from the non-sacrifice of Abraham's son (Delaney 1986). This story is an explicit rejection of the idea that relations with God involve the renunciation of human life, and establishes that a man can enjoy the full fruits of his reproductive endeavours so long as he is entirely obedient to God.

By contrast, the Christian compact with divinity does involve a renunciation of life. Christ was in effect sacrificed to humanity, and men and women are now obliged to embrace a life of self-sacrifice in return. The devaluation of natural sexuality is part of this. It can be argued (Heady 1999) that the identification of divine power with the acceptance of death provides Christians with a way of coping with the fertility-threatening powers of the envious and the moribund. It is customary to refer to the poor (who have particular grounds for envy) and the dead as *biat* – 'blessed' – and to conceptualize one's own struggles in life as sacrifices. The possibility of envy is denied by the universal embracing of the image of renunciation, and the resulting sense of relief is experienced as a divine blessing. Since women are most exposed to the dangerous power of envy, they are most attracted by this paradoxical method of obtaining a sense of safety, which provides another reason for them to endorse the viewpoint of the church.

The different orientations of Islam and Christianity to the natural world seem to be reflected in their core religious symbols – in ways that involve the symbolic use of light. Delaney (1986,1991) does not say much about Anatolian ideas about the forces that govern non-human reproduction, but it would not be surprising if the moon represented some kind of universal generative power, as it does in southern Europe. The cross is certainly *inter alia* a symbol of natural death. So, by placing images of the moon on mosques and crosses on churches, Muslims and Christians are encapsulating this fundamental difference between the two faiths. But in choosing the cross rather than the moon, Christians are not rejecting the symbolic importance of light. The religious images of sacrifice and death in Catholic churches are also sources of symbolic light. The divine power generated by these acts of sacrifice is literally depicted in the form of rays of light – which is consistent with Christian insistence that religious salvation is itself a higher form of life.

LIGHT AND THE DEFINITION OF SOCIAL SPHERES

As well as being associated with natural and divine energy, light in Carnia has connotations of order and social unity. This is true of daylight and the sun. Older people emphasized that they were brought up to fear the dark. I once heard departures referred to metaphorically as *tramonti* – 'sunsets'. It is true as well of the traditional open kitchen hearth – the *fogolar* – round which the family used to sit, which also evokes associations of unity and decency. In fact both *fogolar* and sun combine associations of order and of vital force into images of benign reproduction. Flowers are obvious symbols of the life-giving power of the sun and are also associated with innocence and goodness.

This double meaning of light suggests that it might be possible to create a united community by pooling the reproductive energies of all the individuals who belong to it. This idea is in fact enacted in the *cidulas* ceremony in which the young men throw burning disks down towards the village. These disks, each representing one of the couples they have announced, are lit at a common bonfire, and many other features of the ceremony indicate that it evokes the idea of a sense of village unity based on the sympathetic encouragement of each others' love affairs. Church services and religious processions represent an analogous attempt to build unity by jointly evoking divine energy.

But shared light from one point of view implies darkness from another. The *cidulas* ceremony is based on light, but is held after dark amid various signs of disorder, such as drunkenness and mild obscenity, which would not be publicly acceptable in daylight. In church, and on religious processions, priests dress in bright resplendent robes, which proclaim the power of divine grace. But in non-sacred contexts they indicate their self-sacrificing renunciation of the pleasures of everyday life – and of procreation – by generally wearing dark clothes. Though in one sense these two examples present a contrast, they both show that neither shared reproductive energy nor shared renunciation can bring that combination of order and earthly fertility which is symbolized by the everyday light of the sun.

The Christian identification of religious purity with the renunciation of natural procreation means that at any given moment people have to choose between the two, but that in the long run they need access to both (Christian 1989). So it is not surprising that *cidulas* celebrations are often associated with religious occasions, such as the eve of a saint's day, nor that the proceedings often include some mild mockery of the Church. In effect the symbolism of light helps to define two spheres of social life with distinct criteria of moral legitimacy.

The first of these is the official sphere where religious values reinforce the authority of the old. In this sphere the rhetoric of sacrifice is the dominant way in which moral claims are asserted. It is used to talk about work and the rewards it brings, as well as to justify parental claims to consideration from their children – with the implication that these rights follow from the work parents have done. Indeed, even one of the metaphors used to speak about procreation is economic. The slang word for being pregnant is *compra*, the main meaning of which is 'to buy'. I did not obtain a clear explanation of this expression, but it is consistent with the notion that it is renunciation and the expenditure of resources which provide rights over a child.

The other sphere is the social world of young people. Underlying the symbolism is the notion that this sphere too has its own legitimacy – based on the natural rights of youth and biological vigour. Its ritually marked separation from the sphere of religiously sanctioned parental authority legitimates the idea, which seems to be long-standing, that young people's choice of marriage partners does not concern the older generation. Indeed this is one of the points which is symbolically affirmed by the *cidulas* ceremony. This institutionalized generation gap seems to be absent in Anatolia, where the basic idea, that male sexuality is legitimate so long as it is combined with obedience to authority, provides an ideological basis for the right of fathers to chose marriage partners for their offspring.

THE EQUIVALENCE OF PEOPLE AND LAND

So far, I have analysed the way in which the imagery of light reflects relationships amongst people, and between people and divinity. But one of the most notable features of the imagery is that it also suggests some kind of link between the biological processes affecting people and plants. This can be thought of as an explicit, if partial, formulation of a principle that operates tacitly in other ways as well – namely the equivalence of people and agricultural land.

This equivalence is demonstrated in several ways. The rhetoric of sacrifice which people use to justify parents' claims on their children is also used to establish their moral right to their land. The word for being in charge of people – *comanda* – can also be used to indicate land ownership. Land owned by the family can be referred to as being *in cjasa* – in the house – just like the human members of the family. There is a dangerous magic snake, known as the *codar* – a word which also refers to an implement used in reaping – whose powers seem to embody a resistance to the transfer of life force from land to people in reaping, just as dying people resist the transfer of their life force to those about to take their place. The implicit aggressiveness towards the land involved in reaping used also to be combined with ritual aggression towards neighbouring human communities, embodied in stereotyped name-calling as people from different villages worked their way up the hay meadows on neighbouring slopes. The overall implication is that people have a single system of implicit ideas about relationships involving natural vigour, power and authority, and that these ideas are used in the same way to formulate both rights over people and rights over land.

This conclusion lends support to a very interesting hypothesis of Delaney's about the reason for the stress on endogamy (at both kinship and village level) in Anatolia. Until the 1960s village endogamy was also positively valued in Carnia, and reinforced by ritual, though it did not attain the levels reported by Delaney. Delaney (1991) notes that explanations of endogamy in terms of the need to keep property in the family or community do not work in Anatolia, since inheritance customs would have been enough in themselves to achieve that purpose – another point which appears generally applicable to Carnia as well. Delaney's suggestion is that Anatolians arrange marriages that keep their daughters within the community because they feel that their daughters in some ways *are* fields. Though this may sound rather startling, it would be no more than a specific instance of the equivalence of people and land which, in Carnia at least, is implicitly elaborated in so many ways.

However, this conceptual equivalence between property and personal relationships would only lead to endogamy if property relationships were thought of in a restrictive way, for instance, because of a need to limit access to scarce land. Bloch (1975) has argued persuasively on the basis of Malagasy data that the switch from slash and burn agriculture (in which land is relatively plentiful) to intensive cultivation (in which land is a scarce resource) is indeed accompanied by a movement from exogamy to endogamy. But he concurs with other writers (e.g. Goody 1976) in seeing endogamy as an instrumental way of keeping property within the social group. The Anatolian and Carnian data suggest that this connection needs to be reformulated in terms of the construction of more general mental schemas which make it possible for relationships of ownership and restricted access to be thought about.

CONCLUSIONS

These findings from another monotheistic society lend a good deal of support to Delaney's (1986) analysis, and in particular to her contention that there are detailed correspondences between ideas about procreation and the conceptualization of gender roles, kinship, divinity and property relationships. However, while in Delaney's analysis these relationships always take the form of parallelisms, this is not the case in Carnia, where the relationships involved in religious salvation systematically invert those involved in biological reproduction. Because of this, Delaney's assertion of an innate affinity between monotheism and a male monopoly of the symbolism of legitimate procreation is not supported by the Carnian data.

There are similarly mixed findings in relation to the ideas put forward by Bloch and Parry (1982). A symbolic opposition between natural and divine fertility is certainly present in both Anatolia and Carnia, but in neither case is it treated quite in the way that Bloch and Parry describe. In Anatolia there is, as they would expect, an opposition between divine fertility and the corrupt fertility of women. However, this opposition does not extend to all natural fertility; indeed divinity is symbolically identified with the active, masculine aspect of natural fertility. In Carnia, where divine power is contrasted with all sexual fertility, this is accompanied by veneration of the Virgin Mary – an asexual image of female procreative power – and a general feeling that religion is the affair of women. These divergences from theoretical expectations are explicable in terms of another departure from Bloch and Parry's assumptions. Although in their scheme of things biological reproduction is represented as a manifestation of female productivity, both the Anatolians and the Carnians view it as an assertion of masculine power. Given that biological reproduction is viewed in this way, the divinely inspired denigration of all natural fertility does not provide a suitable ideological basis for patriarchy.

Overall, these findings suggest that more allowance needs to be made for the potential variability of ideas about both natural fertility and relations with divinity. They also suggest that the apparent constants in each theoretical scheme – the existence of symbolic correspondences between different social spheres, and tensions between divine and natural fertility – do not necessarily operate in a way that reinforces masculine power. Any reformulation of these theories will need to pay as much attention to the inherent logic of the symbolic systems as to the purposes to which they are put.

Finally, we come to the question of why these ideas – of natural fertility, divinity and various kinds of social relationship – are so often associated with imagery involving particular manifestations of light. Each of these ideas is symbolically expressed in several ways, among which the imagery of light is only one. So light-based imagery cannot be said to be necessary to convey them. And yet, in Carnia at least, it is pervasive. This pervasiveness suggests that, however they were originally formulated, any ideas about fertility, power or sociability somehow need to be expressed in a way that involves the imagery of light.

Some aspects of the imagery described above suggest reasons why this might be so. One reason is the ability of bright light to capture people's attention. Light may be used to focus attention on a specific point, such as the burning *cidula* disk and the bonfire from which it has come, or on the holy image which is depicted as emitting rays of light. Or light may create a space in which people can discern and interact with each other, as in the case of sunlight or the light from a *fogolar*. Another reason must lie in light's role as a symbol of life force, which is partly due to the fact that sunlight and moonlight are observably associated with some biological processes (though, in the case of the moon, perhaps not as many as people in Carnia believe). I suspect, though I cannot demonstrate, that there may also be something in our physical and psychological make-up which means that we inherently experience light as an energizing force. Even if this is not so, it seems likely that the meanings and perceptions associated with light are sufficiently salient for it to matter that they are deployed in a way which reinforces rather than contradicts other symbolic messages. The symbolism of light is pervasive because light is impossible to ignore.

NOTES

1 Words in *bold italics* are in Friulian, the local language. Italian words are given in ordinary *italics*.
2 Pronounced *macharots*.
3 In fact women do all of the cooking and most of the agricultural work.

CHAPTER 9

THE ESSENCE OF BEING

PROCREATION AND SEXUALITY IN MID-CENTURY MACEDONIA

ILKA THIESSEN

In this paper I discuss the ideas expressed to me by a group of elderly women, in response to my questions about matters of sexuality, conception, childbirth and gender relations. The interviews took place in the region of Skopska Crna Gora in 1995 and the women were born between 1910 and 1925. This paper is part of a larger project about the lives of a group of women who graduated in engineering. My interest in the lives of their grandmothers was necessary to understand the nature of change in socialist and post-socialist Macedonia. Because the women I interviewed lived through immense changes it is not always possible to know what exactly they thought fifty years ago, but I have tried hard to disentangle 'new' ideas from those they grew up with.[1]

Skopska Crna Gora is a mountainous area close to Skopje and the Serbian border. Recently their proximity to the Serbian border has become a political issue among the population of Skopska Crna Gora who like to identify themselves as Serbian, even though they are Macedonian by nationality. Further this area has a reputation for black magic (see Rheubottom 1993). Yet Skopska Crna Gora is also the closest rural area to the city of Skopje, which can be reached by bus in less than an hour. The bus goes three to five times a day, and school children and their parents commute daily to Skopje and back. Those who can afford it prefer to live in Skopje. Education is highly valued by these peasants and it is not seen as positive for the young people to stay behind in the village and continue a peasant's life.

KINSHIP, AFFINITY AND MARITAL RESIDENCE

A family's surname usually suggested descent from a common ancestor in the male line. A patrilineal, exogamous family would also commonly trace its origin to a particular house or household with a specific 'housename' – that of its patron saint. During weddings particularly, frequent reference was made to the kinship groups to which people belonged. Weddings in Macedonia involved each of the two families inviting guests, and it was only at a wedding that the bride and groom might meet all their kin and affines. These kin furnished a network of relationships on which the married couple hoped to draw for support. Otherwise there was little explicit emphasis on affinal relationships. Marriage was usually virilocal, so it was the groom's family which welcomed 'their bride', whereas the bride's family watched 'their daughter' leave. The new daughter-in-law was only slowly integrated into her new household, the group being sensitive to the protection of its boundaries from malign outsiders. Only after about a year was she slowly allowed to leave the transitional role of a 'new daughter' and take up her role as wife (see Rheubottom 1980:244–5). And only when she had become a mother and proved her procreative capabilities to her husband's family did she become fully integrated into the family. She had then secured the continuation of the family and closed the previously open boundaries behind her. Yet women never completely belonged to a family into which they had married: their solidarity could be questioned, their transitionality seen as a threat. Only with this in mind can much of the material to be presented be understood.

COURTSHIP AND MARRIAGE ARRANGEMENT

The age for marriage varied from seventeen to twenty-five. As households were very closed in on themselves, there were not many opportunities for young people to meet. According to Rheubottom's discussion of the *slava* (feast for a patron saint), which highlights openness, peace and community (Rheubottom 1976:25), it was only when household boundaries were lifted that 'strangers could meet.[2] However, even on such occasions, boundaries were still vulnerable and their violation would have had serious consequences. An old woman from Berevo recalled the time when she first met her husband. She was dancing during one of the *slavas* when a young man from a distant village started dancing next to her. She pleaded with him to stop, and when he insisted, her brothers came and beat him up (and then her), and a few days later they had to marry and she had to leave with her new husband to go to his home. From the time he danced beside her until her wedding she did not return to her own home, nor did she contact her family for many years.

Normally however bride and groom were from the same or neighbouring villages, but from a different lineage. Often marriages would be arranged by the families through a matchmaker and bride and groom would first meet in church. Nevertheless, many of the women knew their husbands, at least by sight, as they were often neighbours. When they went to fetch water they risked a glance or two about them, and perhaps caught the eyes of a local boy.

I believe that some of these customs were due to relatively lenient regulation of marriage by State and Church. Todorova (1993:31) writes:

> the relatively subordinate role of the Orthodox church *vis à vis* the state from its very beginning, and, later on, its status as an inferior religion in the Muslim Ottoman Empire, deprived it of the exclusive privileges and influence over the social life of the people enjoyed by the Catholic Church. This, alongside ensuing ideological differences, in turn explains the greater adaptability of the Orthodox church to secular tradition.

My informants had little to say about legal aspects of marriage, and little more about the creation and significance of affines. They were more talkative about the consummation of the marriage as this guaranteed the continuation of the family, unless blocked by infertility.

ENGAGEMENT, MARRIAGE AND SEXUALITY

It was the engagement ceremony which gave a legal character to the relations between a young man and a young woman, and it usually took place only a few days before the wedding itself. The engagement emphasized the social and economic relationship between affines, including negotiations over bridewealth and dowry. Marriage was the moment in life that made men and women into fully social persons as they guaranteed descent group continuity. At the engagement ceremony the bride would receive gifts such as jewellery and gold coins as her personal property. The dowry consisted of clothing, household goods and money; it included communal property of the family she married into, as well as her own personal property, later inherited by her children.

The day of the wedding would then be set, usually a Sunday. It started with the bride's hair being ceremoniously combed and the groom being shaved. The groom's agnates would set out for the bridal home to fetch the bride. At her home the wedding guests would be welcomed and invited for a meal. The groom's agnates would offer presents to the bride's female relatives. When trying to enter the bride's home a fight was enacted, but after she was presented with her wedding shoes the bride would come out and go with her new family to the house where the marriage was to be consummated.

The relationship of a new bride to her husband was difficult to start with. She was in a very vulnerable position in her new household because of her ambiguous position as affine to the groom's agnates. Affinity blurred the boundaries of the family and left the family exposed. The woman new to the group had to gain a position first as wife and then as mother. Rheubottom points out that:

> the bride is immediately incorporated into the work parties of the unmarried women and treated as part of her mother-in-law's conjugal family. If the bride is treated as 'daughter', little is made of her new status as wife. As I have noted, the bond between husband and wife is treated as if it did not exist. Indeed, her husband plays only a small part in the entire wedding celebration' (Rheubottom, 1980:245).

Only after the woman has given birth to her first child do she and her husband become a single unit.

For most women the relationship with their husbands was accompanied by beatings:

> my husband would come back from work (wanting to sleep with her) no matter where, just when he felt like it. Lots of people were living in the house, but he did not care, and when he felt like it, the woman had to do it. Three sisters were living

> in the house with us, as well as the grandmother, and the children, and if I did not want to, he beat me up, always beating me, for everything.
>
> If the husband wanted his wife he would beat her with his stick and I knew I had to go there, so if he was out with the sheep I had to bring him food there and there he would do it, do his job.

All of the women emphasized that the most important thing for a woman was a husband who would not beat her, this is what counted, otherwise any marriage would be fine, because there were children: 'My husband was my neighbour. First I did not like him, but when I got engaged I got used to him and I thought I would love him forever. That's what I tell these young girls, they always talk about love.' And: 'It is hard for the woman. When you know him it is fine, but in our time it was important that he had a house, that he had a goat, and not whether he was a good man and would treat you nicely.'

Another woman told me: 'It is important that he did not beat you. He will like you, he will want you.' The women thought that sex was what men cared about most, and they felt that if they could satisfy a man in this respect, and work hard and raise their children properly, they could have a happy relationship with their husbands. 'That (sex) is what is important for a man. For the woman the children are the most important.' Motherhood strengthened their position as wives.

However, a woman's stronger position as wife paralleled the weakening of the position of her mother-in-law. Her sexuality was a future blessing but also a present threat to her new family and had to be contained. Her sexuality implied that eventually her family would split away from the household, and so represented a diversion of her husband's interest from his parents to his own wife and children. If the incoming bride drew attention to her sexuality, this was seen as a threat to the unity of her husband's family. Women tried to hide their pregnancies from their in-laws for as long as they could, because pregnancy was the ultimate sign of a sexuality that would eventually split her husband's household and would position her at the centre of a new household – that of her husband and their children. (Comments on the shame of a woman's pregnancy and sexuality have to be understood in this light. Signs of sexual maturity in a girl also reminded her natal family of her temporary membership in the family. One woman was so embarrassed when she grew breasts that she hid away from her father; and later when she got her period, she was told by her mother to hide from her father again as he would not welcome the news.)

The roughness of the husband towards his wife in the first years of marriage can be understood in the same way. His solidarity with his family meant he was supposed to show no noticeable interest in his own wife or in her sexuality. If he spoke to her at all in public, he had to be gruff and commanding, displaying little apparent enthusiasm for the marriage bed. This was the public stance, but all my women informants made it clear that their husbands were, in private, intensely interested in sexual relations, and that it was this which legitimated them as wives.

The bride's virginity was important at the consummation of the marriage. If it was discovered that a woman was not a virgin, she was sent back to her own home. When I asked one woman if she was scared to get married I was told that of course she was, as she did not know if she was a virgin. When I inquired why she did not know this, she told me that the groom might sometimes sneak into the bride's room, before the wedding, and then later on the wedding night he might 'discover' that she was not a virgin. The virginity and the procreative capacity of the woman did not belong to her, but to her husband and agnates. As one woman put it: 'Why would a woman no longer be a virgin? Only because of a man, but it is she who gets the blame.' Another woman told me about the advice her aunt gave her, that she should take care that her husband did not put his semen into her, but that first she should live her own life for a year: 'I had no idea what she was talking about, but I told my husband to wait and he respected that. Men know these things, I did not know anything.' This woman was nineteen at the time of her marriage. Only later did women learn to use their procreative capacities for their own ends. For children were seen as a mother's children and constituted her strength.

It became apparent that the women I interviewed saw their own sexuality, not only their procreative capacity, as slowly becoming a source of power over their husbands, whom they portrayed as absolutely addicted to their wives. This emphasis went so far that many of the women stressed that men loved to have sexual intercourse with menstruating women:

> We once went to a mill, my husband and I, and he wanted to be with me – I could not say no because he was beating me, but men did not understand anything. When he wanted it, you were supposed to give it to him and he was not interested in anything else. Now I hear that women do not sleep with their husbands before they have finished menstruating. But whatever, children are always possible, before, after or during menstruation.[3]

Some of the women explained their husbands' interest in sex with their menstruating wives, by their ignorance. One of the women told me: 'We were bleeding and we could not hide it. Men were not scared of it; some even liked a woman especially when she was bleeding.' Five women told me, in one way or an other, that their husbands liked to sleep with them especially during menstruation. One of the women told me: 'Some men are even so crazy that they take you while you are bleeding, some men like you especially then, though other men do not like it, and think it will pollute them.' Another woman told me:

> For the first three months of my marriage I didn't get pregnant, and a cousin started asking why I wasn't pregnant yet. I didn't tell my husband that I was menstruating when he wanted me, but he liked it very much then, and he was wondering why and the next day we went to the field and he wanted it again and again, he liked it very much and then our son was conceived.

She found it very embarrassing to mention how keen her husband was on sex with her.

Most women told me that they did not learn about sexual matters until they married. 'Women talked to each other about these things. We never went to the doctor, we only talked about these things and then we simply did them. God gives what he gives, that's all we knew. Dogs were taken more care of than we were.' Some of the women I talked to had been 'initiated' by some older woman, aunt or neighbour, never by their mother,[4] in what to do after marriage, 'how to lie down and how to do things'. The women told me about their fears, being scared about giving birth, about lying next to their husbands. Some of them told me humorously that later they were running after their husbands (for sex, understood). What they regretted was that their mothers never talked with them about 'being a woman'. They preferred the way their own daughters or daughters-in-law were bringing up their children. They agreed that in 'their time' it was 'a shame' for women to talk about 'things like that', but that men talked about them more easily. They told me that men were taught everything they had to know before they got married by some older men and that women knew nothing.

GOD AND THE RELIGIOUS ELEMENT

Initially all the women insisted that they were ignorant, that they knew nothing, and that they were still primitive. I have met this reaction a number of times with older women in Macedonia. Socialism in Macedonia, it was explained to me, meant breaking with old ways and turning one's back on what had been. Thus, the older generation became the un-educated, un-civilized generation, something these old women had heard many times and had internalized. One 50-year-old woman explained that this was because:

> we went to school and broke with the old ways. We were the new generation, the hope of the country – everything that we left behind was backward and primitive. We were the future, but we also left our parents behind, our mothers who toiled to get us an education. We were the ones then who got educated – we had risen from being cattle.

None of the older women had attended school for more than four years and many felt they were ignorant. Comments such as the following were typical: 'I don't know anything, nothing, what should I tell you, I just know nothing.' Another woman said: 'We were stupid in those days, just like sheep.' A third woman commented: 'My children are all very well educated, but I am living in the old way, and I cannot change now. For them, everything is "known". They know everything.' As one woman told me: 'In our time we were too busy. We did not "think" – we worked in the fields and were content merely if our husbands did not beat us.' Another woman said: 'Now a child of five knows how a baby is made. We were ignorant then, and now things are better. So many children died, in those days.' However, another woman expressed a widespread opinion when she told me that: 'we had nothing ... but still our children were healthy, no matter that they are saying nowadays that we knew nothing and that we did everything wrong'.

One woman commented that: 'if I would have been able to go to school for longer, maybe then I would know something. As it is all I can do is pray.'[5] Later she told me: 'God? People talk about God [laughs] – he has nothing to do with it, it is nature. Nature alone determines everything. My children have had an education.' By saying that her children had an education she implies that they had supported the socialist system, and as such she as the mother 'progressed' with them by denying God.[6] Thus, 'nature' or 'science' had been introduced to my informants as an alternative concept to God. They said, 'God decides this, and it is nature.' When I asked the women what the moment of birth meant to them one woman told me: 'We did not ask ourselves where life came from as the "new' people do now.[7] In those days we thought that God gives life, and God takes life away. Nobody said that a man or a woman could make life.' Procreation for these older women then was seen as historically differentiated. Statements about 'in our time' and 'today' are differentiated by life given by God and life given by society. The idea behind this is that socialism introduced agency into the life of individuals. The consummation of marriage for these women was a relationship not between men and women, not between families, but a relationship between them and something higher that defied definition.

They all emphasized that today things are different, but that in the past God gave things and took them away. One woman told me that: 'When you give birth you will know all these things. Nowadays there are two Gods. In the hospital they can give injections, but the babies are still the same.' Thus, the power of medicine and science, which has played a predominant role in socialist society, is referred to as 'another' or 'second' god, a notion repeated in several interviews. They believed themselves to be very much at the mercy of God, of evil spells and evil spirits, and of nature. All of them were proud of how they had managed to bring up their children. One woman really wanted to ask God why he made decisions the way he did, but then sighed and said that she was too stupid to even try to understand God.

All the women mentioned God as being responsible for the

'give and take' of human reproduction. However, they argued with him only in the sense that he was responsible for the uncertainties. They could seek his help, but he alone would decide whether or not to help. Village women everywhere in Macedonia peeled saints' eyes from paintings on church walls, and boiled the peeling in water, as the resulting fluid had healing effects. In the same way women would boil a cross in water or would ask the priest to give them some baptismal-font water to mix with their baby's bathwater to protect it from illness and black magic. Evil spirits and the church were battling against each other, and the women tried to influence the outcome as best they could.

They agreed that it was not good if women could not have children: 'But you cannot do anything about it. Nobody is to blame – it is simply God's will.' They felt they had no influence over this matter. Infertility was not caused by evil spirits, but was the will of God and God could not be influenced. The midwife's task lay more in helping the women to protect themselves from spells than to assist medically: 'The midwife told me to tell nobody when I was giving birth so that nothing bad could happen to me ... but if I sensed that someone knew I would have had to go over the person three times, so I would have no trouble.' The idiom of 'going over a person three times', the woman told me, meant literally stepping over a person three times. The best time to do this would have been when that person was asleep. She added that this was difficult to do and one could still resort to other means. The underlying idea was to distract a potentially jealous person. Three is an auspicious number in Macedonia; for example, to greet a person one should give three kisses on the cheek. These three kisses are for God, his Son, and the Holy Spirit.

Religious symbolism played an important role in giving birth. One of the women told me that the midwife had given her a towel. Her labour was very painful and it went on for days, during which time she 'made wooden things break',[8] but when she thought of the towel and that she would take it to church: 'the baby came out just like this, as if someone pulled it away from me'. The towel became the connection between her newborn baby and the church. The child was pulled out of her as if it were holding onto the towel. From all the accounts it appears that the church played a major role for these older women in functions of 'giving birth' and 'managing death', spiritually and practically. Today they are faced with the world inhabited by their children and grandchildren in which those tasks are taken over by medicine and science. They are told by their children that they had been living in ignorance and that today society has taken control of such fundamental issues as birth and death. However, my informants seemed unconvinced. Their telling me that they are ignorant and do not know anything is more mimicking the official party line. Often, as I mentioned earlier, they told me that despite all the odds they had been able to raise healthy children. And some saw that society today has as much control over life and death as they had – only with different kinds of 'ritual' and in different guise.

INSEMINATION AND THE CREATION OF THE CHILD

Procreation, or better, 'making children', had specific aspects for the women I interviewed. Women would describe how they slept with their husbands; what would determine if it would be a boy/child (the two words are the same in Macedonian) or a girl; what determines the baby's appearance; and in what way the children were formed into people. All emphasized that children, boys and girls, are more important for a woman than a man as they will be the ones who take care of her in her old age. They were not all clear about what exactly happened biologically but had similar ideas. The most common explanation the women gave was similar to: 'you sleep with your husband and he puts his semen into you and if you do this while you are bleeding you will have a daughter, otherwise it will be a child (boy). It is God's will if a child results.'

Blood and semen are similar substances which most of all indicate strength. They are not substances that 'create' a child, as only God creates, but they give strength. When these are joined successfully a child will be born. One woman explained that semen is similar to the blood of menstruating women: 'If the woman were to have no semen then there is no child, she cannot give birth. The woman bleeds inside to feed the child. If she bleeds outside she has no child.' Blood and semen also come to stand for sexual desire. Sexual desire is a form of strength. Women's strength was not supposed to be channelled into sexual desire but into their love for their children and family. A woman who demonstrated her sexual desire was often seen 'as a man'.

Women are seen as nurturing the baby, giving the baby their life force in the form of blood (*krv*). Thus they told me that: 'if the woman is strong, the baby is strong, so it does have to do with her'. But one of the women told me that she found it strange that weak women would always have the strongest children, whereas the strong women have weak and sickly children. I believe this to be related to the idea that a strong woman would use up all the nurturing blood herself and have nothing left for her baby, whereas the weak woman would give all her strength to her child. *Krv* (blood) was important in other respects too. If the child looks similar to its family this is a result of the blood. Some women repeated what the priest had told them, that at marriage the two bloods were 'joined'. When I asked the women what semen was or where it came from they told me that the semen came from God, and menstrual blood and semen both go into the child. 'Men and women cannot be without each other.'

All the women had similar answers to the question of what determines if a baby is a boy or a girl. If the woman was strong and more powerful than her husband (at the moment of intercourse – something which made a few of the women giggle, then the woman would give birth to a girl. They told me that if the child looked like the mother, the mother had been stronger (in a physical sense) as well, and added that in this case people would laugh at the father. One woman suggested that if a couple had only boys, it showed that the husband was stronger than his wife. Another said that in the uterus the semen of man and woman fight and the one that is stronger determines if it will be a boy or a girl.[9] Most women said that either girl babies or especially strong boy babies were conceived while the woman was menstruating. Such 'explanations' varied from woman to woman. One woman told me that before and after menstruation the woman would conceive a boy (and conceive a girl while menstruating). I was also told that, if one wanted a boy, the woman should sleep with her husband one week before menstruation and then the boy would be especially strong.

In these accounts the concept of strength is predominant. Male and female substances do not create the child or its sex, but it is the relative strength of male and female substances that determine the child physically and morally, and later further shape it. Blood is the strength of the mother, semen the strength of the father. Only one woman told me that conception cannot occur while the woman is menstruating. Neither male semen alone, nor menstrual blood alone, creates the child or determines its sex. Many of the women told me that it required several acts of intercourse to make a child.

INFERTILITY, WOMEN'S STRATEGIES AND THE EVIL EYE

To remain unmarried, or to be married but barren, was terrible, the women agreed. 'If you have not given birth you are not a woman' was the sentiment. This was the reason a woman got married. Some women told me that being able to give birth was related to 'having the will'. After giving birth they would 'wash their babies with ashes' so they would not fall victim to the evil eye, meaning their babies would become undesirable to others, because to have children meant to have people envy them. Children were the greatest treasure a family could have.

All the women thought that one could not really do anything when someone was infertile (even though some of the women told me that it depended only on one's will). As I have already noted the general condition of barrenness was seen as the will of God. 'When God wants to give a child he will give you one, it is not up to you. Now young people think they can do everything, that it is they who "decide" how many children they have. They replace God, but I do not understand with what.' Most of them agreed, not only that infertility could also be the husband's fault, but more that it was most commonly his fault: 'If nothing comes it is not the woman's fault. If God wants it, whenever you have sex with a man you can have children. If you do not want a child you should stay away from each other.'

It is possible that, in recognizing that barrenness could be a male problem, my informants were projecting 'new' scientific knowledge back into their early lives. A few accounts, however, did suggest that people really had been aware of male infertility. All of the women interviewed mentioned that it could very well be the husband's problem. 'Ah, the husband would marry somebody else and then this woman wouldn't have children either – is that not proof enough?' Asked if men would remarry such divorced women, they agreed that they would:

> it was difficult to obtain a woman and it cost a lot of money. Men had to pay for us – it was difficult for them. First they

> bought a house, then a woman ... Before marriage a woman was not valued at all, not kept well until she married. Then she was treasured, but then, too, he might beat her up. Before (the marriage) he would send people, money, bags ... Yes, parents would sell a daughter and they would not ask her who she wanted.

I found most intriguing personally what the women told me about a specific female conspiracy in one case of infertility. One woman told me this:

> When I was young you could not go to the doctor to see who was not able to make a child. The old women then, when they saw that there was a hopeless case, would come together and take the woman to another man so she would get pregnant. Nobody was supposed to know this, not the husband, not anybody, so the husband would think it was his child ... Even if the people then were illiterate and simple they knew how to keep secrets, so the lie would not fall apart. When the child would not look like his mother or father then the old women would say: 'oh, he looks like his uncle nine generations [lit. "belts"] ago', yes, then the old women would say: 'oh, the baby looks just like his uncle'. In those days men trusted the old women, and that's how they could arrange such things.

Such accounts throw new light on the alleged powerlessness of women. One has to take into account that when the women remember that they were beaten and completely subject to the will of their husbands, they are often recalling their first years of marriage. While I was sitting with them and chatting, it was the husband who brought us tea and who was tenderly shushed. Certainly, in later years their positions in their households had improved and, as wives and mothers, they had far more control over their lives than at the beginning of their marriages.

BIRTH SPACING AND MALE-FEMALE RELATIONS

Without children a woman had no power at all. Too many children, however, meant poverty. There was not always enough land to feed extra hungry mouths. Regulating fertility thus became important.[10] Generally only two methods of doing this were mentioned in the interviews. One was abstinence, which the women claimed was difficult for the men to observe, and the other was *coitus interruptus*. Regulating fertility was described as a man's responsibility.

Abortion was legal in socialist Yugoslavia, and continues to be so in today's Macedonian Republic. In other interviews younger women told me quite frankly that they had had very many (up to nine) abortions in their lives. One woman, when asked why she had had so many abortions, told me that she did not know what else to do and that her doctor promoted abortions, 'as it was cleaning me inside'. Something similar was said about actual childbirth: 'Having children makes you cleaner – it fulfils you.' But the old women I interviewed in Skopska Crna Gora never mentioned abortion as a practice they had employed in their youth. One woman in the village told me: 'We did not take such care, we just took what we got and did not think of what we could have done, as my daughters do now.' It seems that infant mortality was so high that abortions were not 'needed'. What was seen as important was the spacing of pregnancies.

FOETAL DEVELOPMENT AND COMPLICATIONS

If the women agreed that the birth of a boy or a girl depended on the relative strengths of father and mother, as discussed above, they also claimed that if the baby's face was similar to that of the mother, she was seen as stronger than her husband. However, some of the women also emphasized that the baby had only one blood, that of its parents, as husband and wife were one blood and their blood mixed:

> That's the reason the priest chants at the wedding, husband and wife are one blood now and that's why sometimes the daughter looks like the father, it is the blood. The mother has been stronger, but they are of the same blood. This is why the girl looks like the father or the baby looks like the mother. They are all of one blood.

Or, I was told, that usually people would say that the son looks like his father and the daughter looks like her mother and sometimes they would look like some other relative, but God would decide this; it is nature. Sometimes I was told the mother would be troubled because the child did not look like either its father or mother and then people thought the woman must have been with another man. One woman told me: 'Today people know about hormones that decide if you have a daughter or a son, but then we did not know, and we thought it was the men who were to blame if they sometimes father only boys or only girls.' If a child resembled its mother she had either looked, while sleeping with her husband, in the direction of her natal home, or she had turned towards it at her wedding; her children then would have her family features.

I was also told that if the father was a thief the son would be a thief, as this was determined by blood as well. All women agreed, though, that the blood was a joint matter and that a child would always have something from the father as well as from the mother. In addition I was told that when the father drank a lot, he had no strength and could not do anything; his semen would be weak. Cold and warmth also influenced the quality of the semen. Hot weather was supposed to be better for semen, as I was told by one woman: 'it is because it is the time when the fields grow. God wants it like this.'

Women stressed how many children died in the past. None of the women I interviewed had more than three living children. They told me that: 'today things are different, today you have injections against death'. One woman mentioned that many children died from measles and that they could not do anything about it because the doctor was far away. If they wanted to bring their child to the doctor they had to tie it on their back in a cradle and walk for hours as there was no other means of transportation. Thus, it seems that survival of both mother and child was directly related to the mother's health. The 40 days of the *leunka* (see below) were, I believe, seen as a time to preserve the woman's health and take special care for the child. Thus, I believe, the 40 days were related less to concepts of pollution than to the protection of the mother.

BIRTH AND MIDWIVES

I started my interviews by asking women about when they gave birth. They felt at ease with this question and told me about it eagerly and proudly. 'Now you give birth in bed, then we had only hay like the cows. Yes, that's how Mary gave birth, that's how we knew how to give birth.' It was not at all easy for them, but it was for all of them an extraordinary task they managed by themselves.

> The moment of giving birth I remember as if it were now. It was very difficult. We were four people at home and we had eight workers and I had to make food for them. We had no beds, we were sleeping on the floor. But birth then was such happiness and joy. It is what the woman can give to the family, but you could not afford to feel anything special or important, we were so many at home and everybody had to work.

Some were all alone; some had a midwife with them who would help and advise them. Nearly all the women mentioned the secrecy surrounding birth so as not to attract evil spirits and also because of the shame of possibly being seen naked. They were burdened by such secrecy, as they themselves did not really know what was happening. Generally they described giving birth as the moment when they started to have pain.

> Then when I gave birth we opened up all the doors from the house, from the cupboards, from everywhere, the closets and everywhere, so the uterus would open – it would open easier then. I was kneeling down, like a chicken, that's how we used to do it, like a chicken laying eggs.

After birth the baby was swaddled completely for 40 days. Its arms and legs would be bound so they would become straight. Children would be kept like this for a whole year. The women mentioned how beautiful the children were then, and that 'now men and women are like dwarfs, then people were big and nice, because they were swaddled'. They also thought that today there were more people with defects because they were not bound. There was another way of forming the child; I was told that soon after the birth the midwife (*babica)* would massage the baby's face, and particularly the nose to give them a good shape.

After giving birth, the woman cut the umbilical cord herself, and the midwife came and announced the birth. All of the women agreed that the greatest danger for a woman giving birth was bad spells that might have been put on her. Past evil deeds could also have caused problems, and they agreed that this was not so nowadays. Spells, they claimed, were not dangerous for the women today. One woman told me she was keeping some of the *lactovit* (milk substitute) her granddaughter was fed with as a memento: 'We had nothing like this, in our time we did not observe any real rules, but we did what we could.' If the baby was not well the women took it first to the *babica* and then to the priest or to the doctor, depending on whether they could afford a doctor. The *babica* would call the spirits and cure the child.

> There were many women doing such things those days, they would dance around the fire and spit water on you. They were probably praying to God and we thought they knew so much. They were doing strange things, moving glasses and they put shells in the water. Now we know that you can get these shells everywhere from the sea-side but then we did not know. It was such a common thing and we paid out money for such things.

Some women were thought to look at the child with envy. A woman would say how beautiful the baby was and how healthy, but with the envy from her eyes she would put a spell on it. When such a person left, the child had to be wiggled on a chair to shake off the spell. Women would offer a lock of their own hair on a first visit to a new-born child, just in case they were unconsciously envious, so that they could not hurt the baby. The mother would take the hair of the visiting and potentially envious woman, and put it on the fire while holding the child over it in order to remove any spell.

THE POST-PARTUM CONDITION: LEUNKATA

All the women had been accorded a special status for the 40 days after birth when the new mother was called *leunka*, or *leunkata* or *rodelkata*.[11] 'For the first 40 days the families would take more care of their *leunkata*, so they gave her more food. She had lost blood so she had to regain her strength, but after 40 days nobody paid her special attention anymore.' All my informants had observed some of the *leunka* regulations, mostly the avoidance of church ground. The women mentioned pollution only in respect of this avoidance: 'For 40 days the *leunka* could not go into a church. She had to become clean first.' One woman told me that the *leunka* was supposed to hide and relatives were not allowed to see the mother because it was shameful.

Depending on the season, women who had recently given birth would have to return to work in the fields. However, during the 40 days of the *leunka* condition they were not supposed to be out after sunset, because it was believed that otherwise the maternal milk would dry up. A few women mentioned that the *leunkata* should not drink any water because her stomach would swell up, but she should drink wine because that was good for the milk. The woman had also to wear a red thread around her right hand. She was not supposed to meet any other *Leunka* who had given birth in the same week, lest one of their children should die. However, when such a meeting could not be avoided, the women had to exchange rings. During these 40 days none of the women were allowed to enter church nor were they allowed to sleep with their husbands, for the sake of their own health, some women thought (though I was told that the husbands did not really care about this). After the fortieth day they would go with their child to church and pray. Other people would go with them to ask the priest for baptismal water. The *leunka* would send him a bottle of water, the priest would pray over the water and chant, then he would return it. The *leunka* would put a little of the water into the baby's bathwater, and such water would ensure she would have enough milk.

Before the sixth week was over, the family and the prospective godfather would take the baby into the church. The godfather gave the child a name – the mother still could not be present in church[12] Then children ran to her and told her the name of the child (and they would then get some money for telling this news to the mother). When I asked why the mother was not allowed to go I was told: 'she is still a *leunka*; maybe she is more vulnerable and her milk could be cursed'. I believe from these and similar comments that the women refused to see themselves as polluting, but were certainly in a condition of vulnerability, as was their child.

WOMEN AS MOTHERS

I mentioned above that the responsibility for forming the child's personality and giving it an education lay in women's hands. In most of my interviews I could sense this special relationship between mothers and children or grandmothers and grandchildren, while men did not seem to be included in this emotional bonding, but operated more in the 'political' sector of kinship I am not suggesting that fathers did not love their children; however, emotionally there appeared to be greater bonding between mothers and children. This placed a lot of responsibility on women.[13]

A few of my informants would agree with what one of the old ladies said: 'It is too bad that you have to sleep with a man to have children. Children are a woman's riches, the only thing that gets her recognition.' Children were seen as 'mother's children'. The father participated only with a small moment of personal joy, but as all the women stated, it is the mother who nurtures her child, first in the nine months she carries it, with her pain, and after birth for the rest of her life. Some women pointed out that it was they who organized their children to go to school and university; with their hard labour they made it possible for their children to live a different life to the one they had lived. This reinforces all the other information I collected over the years: mothers have a fundamental role in bringing up their children[14]

CONCLUSION

In the preceding pages I have attempted to find the essence of procreative being, or more, the understanding of it amongst a small group of Skopska Crna Gora women. What I found is mirrored by an ambivalence Juliet du Boulay pointed out in her 1986 discussion on: 'Women – images of their nature and destiny in rural Greece'. Du Boulay sees this ambivalence arising through the opposing imagery of the two female prototypes: Eve who, through sin, has caused mankind to fall, and Mary, the mother of God. One is seen as inferior and impure; the latter is seen as the upholder of religion and tradition, the ultimate mother. In Christian religion such ambivalence is resolved by assigning the image of Eve and the image of Mary to different phases in the development of womanhood. Eve is the seductive, unmarried, unproductive woman, whereas Mary becomes the image of the all-holy mother, a symbolic understanding widespread in eastern European societies and in the Mediterranean. Thus, reproduction becomes the ultimate goal of every woman and is seen as her power base. However, in contrast to Delaney's discussion, in Skopska Crna Gora children are not 'given as a present' by men to women, but are given by God. However, God is not the ultimate male in the sense that Mary is the ultimate mother and woman. In contrast to God, Mary has a human origin and Jesus is pictured as her child. Mankind is thus distinct from God and men are not equal to God. Women and men in Skopska Crna Gora are fulfilling the plan of God; God for them is the essence of being. In this world it is the task of men and women equally to contribute to the passing of essence of being onto future generations. The essence itself, the life force, lies in the blood of women and men. When the priest joins the blood of wife and husband he gives his blessing to the passing on of joined life force. What men and women are giving to life is their strength; only united do they have the strength to pass on life. Such gendered strengths are complementary. However, as du Boulay pointed out for Greece (1986:147):

> marriage used to be virilocal – it being, until very recent times, the custom for any sons to bring their wives into the parental household, to live as a joint family until such time as it was thought that the inheritance should be divided and the various families go to live separately. When this happened, it fell to the lot of one son, usually the youngest, to stay in the familial house with the now ageing parents, to look after them, and, after their death, to inherit the house and a significant part of the land and appurtenances of the farm.

As this holds for Macedonia too, it can be concluded:

> This situation thus created an obvious fault line between the mother-in-law and the bride (or brides) who came into her house; for while she was happy for her son to marry and to give her grandchildren, and happy also to have a younger woman in her house to work under her direction, she was also aware that the incoming woman would be a threat, both through her ability to take over the affection of her son and in the fact that by her very youth and strength she was in an ultimately victorious position, waiting only for the older woman to die before she would in turn become the mistress of the house. (Du Boulay 1986:147).

So it was in this vulnerable position towards her mother-in-law, whose solidarity the young woman could not count on, that the young woman felt insecure. She was beaten by her husband, feared him and felt worthless. This however gradually changed over the years, mostly through her ability to bear children. Being a mother slowly transformed the young bride into the centre of the house; in old age with grandchildren, her influence extended and was recognized by her husband. Beating his wife showed that the husband kept his solidarity with his parents and it proved his strength to his wife, a strength she did not necessarily dislike as it showed the strength of his blood, a strength the woman needed to have a healthy child. It is up to a woman's strength, up to her 'will', to nurture and raise her children and to pass on the essence of life. Nevertheless, for this to be possible, it is irrevocably linked to her husband's strength; and only together can they pass on life. As such the question is not 'who creates life?': the semen of men or the woman's contribution to the child through some other substance? It is not a matter of substance, but only a matter of relative strength.

NOTES

This research was carried out under the direction of Professor Peter Loizos, with funds from the LSE Geography and Anthropology Research Division, for whose support I am grateful.

1 One setback in some of my interviews was a woman who came to 'control' what was said. I was not able to determine her role and learned only that she was the milk mother of my friend's father, his aunt. She would just come into the house, sit down and listen. She intervened when the topic turned to magic – she insisted that there was nothing like black magic, that this was all nonsense. The women interviewed would then be much more careful in what they told me and in one case I had to stop the interview because the interviewed woman suddenly became very silent. Dina in Skopje who had left the village because of black magic refused to talk about this woman. However, as my interviews were about birth, baby care and 'making children' we only touched slightly on the topic of black magic.

2 'It is important to add that most of the guests are not literally 'strangers' to the host. Indeed most of the guests are kin, affines, neighbours, and close friends. . . .' (Rheubottom 1976:24).

3 Later on this woman explained that children can be made any time, even if the woman was menstruating.

4 The relationship between mother and daughter is a relationship of intimacy that nevertheless emphasizes generational hierarchy. A mother will not treat her daughter in a woman-to-woman manner,

but always in the power structure of mother to child. In every family, in every house it is the mother, the prototype being the 'mother of God', who takes the central position.

5 She is referring to socialist discourse on peasant ignorance. A stage of slavery had kept them in this ignorance and it was their children who were freed from this ignorance through the socialist party. Nearly all the old people would state this with a tone of bitterness, feeling that their children had left them behind and were looking down on them for the life they had led.

6 In many families, generational conflict took the form of the parents following socialist ideology and the grandparents trying to circumvent them by secretly having their grandchildren baptized.

7 In Macedonia there is a specific concept of 'new' people. Either these are young/socialist-, or today young/entrepreneur-like.

8 She refers to her holding onto bed, chair and table while giving birth and breaking the actual bed frame.

9 To my question of what they meant by 'stronger' I did not get any answer but only more giggles, but as suggested elsewhere they were probably talking about intercourse position – the woman being 'stronger' means 'above' the man.

10 I asked them what the ideal number of children would be for them. They told me that many children were good as they could help in the fields and would support them when they were old, but that probably too many children (more than six) would mean great poverty for the family. However, they told me that there were never that many surviving children. Many children died very young or later in the war.

11 In Macedonian the term *rod* denotes 'to give birth to', or, *rodena* means 'given birth to': *ja sum rodena* = 'I am born' (where/when). *Roditeli* are parents. *Rod* also means gender, but primarily it has the meaning of kin. *Leunka* is not found in the standard English/Macedonian dictionary and the women did not know where the term came from, but they all used it specifically for the first 40 days of motherhood.

12 It is important to note here that in Macedonia it is much more the name day that is celebrated and not the birthday. Birthday is more something that is 'copied' from western TV. Nevertheless there are a few people who do not have traditional names and people go through some pain to find the similarly named patron. Name patrons are mostly men (except Maria, Ana, etc.) and married women were often addressed by their husband's first name. The wife of Mite would be Mitica, or the wife of Mile would be Milica.

13 Marriage means, for women, having children, while for men it is primarily about economic links between affines. Men are supposed to help the family of their wives, but they also gain a 'connection' they can utilize.

14 Today, at divorce, children stay with their mothers most of time.

CHAPTER 10

PROCREATION METAPHORS IN RURAL GREECE

CULTIVATING, BREAD-MAKING, WEAVING*

THEODORE PARADELLIS

In this paper I will first briefly refer to some material concerning beliefs on sexuality and procreation in late nineteenth- and early twentieth-century Greece, and then explore three birth metaphors used explicitly or implicitly concluding with a short theoretical comment on metaphor and models. The paper is part of a larger work dealing with the symbolic construction of procreation, pregnancy and birth, where I focus on meanings, ideas, rituals and values as they are portrayed in archival material. My sources are mostly folkloric, collected (with few exceptions) between the second half of the nineteenth century and the 1940s.[1] An interesting aspect of the folkloric materials is that they show considerable consistency in the way they classify and record the material (something like the famous 'Notes and Queries' in British anthropology[2]. Although the period in which these sources were collected extends at least to over a century, we have more or less the same categories, the same way of approaching the 'reality' recorded. I should also add that the informants are mostly women.

In a folk version of the Genesis story, before tasting the fruit (fig) Adam and Eve 'did not know how to make children'. After they ate it, the hair covering their bodies fell of. Seeing they were nude, they felt shame towards one another: 'They joined their thighs, and put their hands over their heads ... and they joined their armpits. At the point where they had joined there was still hair left over, the rest fell off.' God expelled them from Paradise, after he put a curse on Adam: 'You will labour, arduously day and night, and you will be barely able to feed your children.'

And to Eve he said, 'You will bear children in pain, feed them with your breasts for several years, you will work and struggle, and your daily work will be damned.' Hence, man attends to the earth constantly ('he is made of soil'), and woman, who 'comes from man, and is not made of soil' looks after her man, while her work doesn't count' (Megas 1929). The general idea is that 'women are Eves', 'women have no faith', they are a constant threat as 'the woman deceived the Devil', 'you can confine neither the wind nor a woman', 'women have plenty of hair but hardly any brains', and 'women are all about dancing, and fucking'. 'Woman is the wildest animal of all', 'her hair has more drawing power than a horse-drawn cart' (Politis 1899–1902;II,83 and VI:249 ff; ILLA s.v. *'gynaika'* (woman); also Campbell 1964:276–7 and du Boulay 1974:101–5).

Before examining the three main birth metaphors used in the context of Greek culture, we must consider a few details regarding the two basic substances that contribute to the creation of new life. *Sperm* is supposedly produced in the spinal cord and is responsible for conception, an idea we also find in Hippocrates and his tradition. Sexual relations upset man's work, they are prohibited on holy days, and excessive sexual activity is said to cause damage to the spinal cord (Kouzis nd.: 820; Argenti and Rose, 1949:408–9; Onians 1951:182; Campbell 1964:276–7; Blum and Blum 1965:115; Heritier-Augé 1985:119–21; Psychogios 1989:34). Beliefs concerning the evils of masturbation are suggestive. It leads to the destruction 'of the most precious body fluid' (sperm), 'one measure of sperm is worth forty measures of blood, and its strength is equal'. The effects of masturbation on the body ('according to physicians and doctors') include a progressive weakening of the organism, of sight and intelligence, the loss 'of all virility of body and of soul as [men] become womanly', 'nocturnal ejaculation ... on account of the dilation of the sperm ducts', and premature old age generally (Pyrros 1831 I:42; Pedalion [1800]1976:704–6; see also Brandes 1981:226; McGilvray 1999:82,63; Laqueur 1990:46–7; Loizos and Papataxiarchis 1991:227).

The heart represents the seat of emotion and life, and it contains *blood.* Blood appears to be a live substance, which 'boils', 'bubbles', 'heats up', 'seeks revenge', 'attracts (kinship)', 'cannot become water', its lines follow those of kinship, it is hot or cold, it may mix with other blood and then new life will be created. Blood is thought to be transmitted from parents to children, and to constitute parental property (Politics, I, 350 ff; Campbell 1964:131–2; Kouzis n.d.:820; ILLA s.v. *'aima'* (blood)). Menstrual blood is especially potent, and it is used in love magic. A mother keeps signs of her daughter's first menstrual blood until she reaches marriage age. Then she gives it to the groom to whom they have 'taken a fancy', and he 'becomes mad with desire for her'. On the other hand, men use sperm dried in the sun as a love potion (Megas 1941–2:110; Blum and Blum 1970:131–2; Koukoules 1957:524; Frangaki 1978:33; Psychogios 1989:45–6). A menstruating woman is 'disorderly' (*atsali*), 'polluted', and 'polluting' (*magarismeni*). She must not offer the food she has cooked to the church, for fear of pollution. She could not attend church, receive Holy Communion, touch wine and brine for they will go bad, she should not go near vines, beehives and grain, she should not milk the animals. (ILLA s.v. 'aima' (blood); Campbell 1964:31; Blum and Blum 1967:34, 138; Michailides–Nouaros 1969:184; Danforth 1989:197–8; see also Gélis 1984:35; Buckley and Gottlieb 1988). However, menstrual blood has positive connotations of fertility, and this is evident from its use in love magic. Delayed menstruation and leucorrhoea (white blood) caused severe anxiety. They could be corrected by draining blood from the feet at the time of the new moon, by hot baths, by rue compresses, or by the ingestion of rust, red pepper or red wine with cherry tree root. Menstruation is a necessary prerequisite for childbirth. However, the blood, whose regular appearance is beyond control, in the context of marriage also represents something contrasting to childbirth, i.e. non-conception, no new life, sexuality without motherhood. Thus, many of the herbs used to facilitate menstruation are also used to facilitate abortion, or as aphrodisiacs: rue, parsley, celery, laurel and one herb characteristically called 'killer', or 'killer weed', because it moves the blood' (Pyrros 1831:I 34, II:201; Agapios 1850:147; Saranti-Stamouli 1938:197–8; Megas 1941:167; Frangaki 1978:33; Khaviara-Karachaliou 1993:47–8, 348, 381, 485).

The foetus feeds on menstrual blood. Educated medical theory suggests something similar.

> 'When the man's sperm enters via the lower hole into the woman's uterus, and goes through her tubes to her ovaries, then those eggs, wet and warm, separate each into two and

> through the tubes, they enter the uterus, whether they plant themselves, and suck and suckle the menstrual blood. As these eggs feed there, they enliven the foetus in the women's uterus, and they make it grow'. (Pyrros 1831:I 298).

Another prevalent belief is that those women who experience unusual pains during their periods will not bear children (Frangaki 1978:33). In other words, pain belongs to childbirth and not to menstruation, and the reversal of this relation leads to childlessness.

Menstrual blood is not absolutely dangerous or polluting. Rather it is in the context of processes and substances whose meaning is contrary, and their effect is cosmologically opposite. Thus, menstrual blood must be kept away from various things, except under controlled conditions. For example, the presence of menstrual blood is negative in the context of processes of growth, birth, creation, and transformation in general. Also, it is inconceivable that baked offerings taken to church or Holy Communion should come into any contact with menstrual blood or menstruating women. If this were to happen, the consequences would be dreadful, as God is the only one within whose power it is to 'unite the dissimilar and mix the unmixable' (Kritopoulos, 1893:299). In contrast, after the menopause women may approach the altar. More generally, the church sanctuary must be protected from the infiltration of all bodily substances.

According to the Church 'neither lawful union, nor the blood of childbirth, nor nocturnal ejaculation may pollute man's nature'. However, the Church forbids a menstruating woman from receiving Holy Communion or coming near the altar, for she is polluting and dirty. The reasons, or rather, the rationalizations, suggested by the Church are: (a) that men detest all they consider unclean and abominable 'whatever nature excretes as useless through the orifices of the body' (ear wax, mucus, phlegm, urine, excrement and menstrual blood) – which brings to mind the theory of Mary Douglas (1966); (b) that 'God educates men through bodily processes', if these involuntary processes are unclean, 'all the more so are the sins which they commit consciously' a case of redundancy, as the argument purports to explain why 'the natural is unclean'; and (c) that God declares menstruation unclean, 'in order to prevent men from coming into contact with women who are menstruating, for the benefit of the children yet to be born. Because the children who are conceived and fed on such rotten, useless and polluted blood substances ... become weaker in nature ... they get leprosy and they lack limbs' (Pedalion [1800] 1976:547–8; see also Koukoules 1957:41, 523–4; Handman 1980:118).

WILD AND DOMESTICATED FERTILITY

In Greece, fertility in women is understood and expressed principally through the metaphoric conceptual schema of vegetal or plant fertility and reproduction. To be more precise, it is conceived as 'domesticated' plant fertility rather than the uncontrolled fertility of 'wild' nature. When fertility is linked to wildness, this relationship is mediated by symbolic or ritual acts which somehow tame this energy and channel it in a legitimate and moral direction: childbearing in wedlock. But non-legitimate sexuality – namely, extramarital sexual activity – runs counter to fertility, or is associated with a morbid form of fertility leading to teratogenesis, miscarriage, premature death of the newly-born baby or the infant (Frangaki 1969:80, 1978:34). This also happens if husband and wife have sex at times of great religious ceremonies. This ideological framework becomes a self-fulfilling prophecy, since an illegitimate child is given birth to in secret somewhere in the wilderness, as in a traditional song: 'I was cheated, I was seduced, he has dishonoured me.../Which mountain should I climb so that I may give birth to my child/my midwife will be the partridge and my servant will be the eagle'; or once the child is born: 'she carried it off in her apron to throw it over the cliff' (Theros 1951:185). Furthermore, in general it is the *kopello* or *kopeliaro* or the *bastardou* i.e. 'bearer of a bastard' who is considered responsible for the hailstorms which destroy the vineyards and sickness of animals and men; the unmarried mother is believed, that is, to evoke evil (Karapatakis 1979:36–8).

Indeed the word *agrio*, that is 'wild', signifies the undomesticated, untamed, fierce (as in ferocious beast) when referring to animate beings; untiled, self-propagating (as in wild vine), uncultivated, waste land (wilderness, wild mountains) when referring to the inanimate. However, more generally, it implies that which arouses emotions of fear or turmoil, whether it is the *agrio mati* i.e. 'a fierce eye' or 'wild look in one's eye', *agrios kairos*, 'wild weather' or *agria thalassa*, 'raging of the sea', or an *agria* moment in time as in *agria mesanikta* i.e. 'in the dead of night'. It is sometimes used, however, to imply that which is unripe, raw, premature (lacking) and also the excessive and particularly powerful such as *agrios ponos*, 'severe/unbearable pain', *agrio pathos* meaning 'raging desire/uncontrolled passion', and so forth (Papazaphiropoulos 1887:372–3; Politis 1931:72–4; Saranti-Stamouli 1937:353, 1952:177; ILLA s.v. *'agrios'* (wild).

Mainly forces hostile towards man dwell in the wild, although they often approach and lurk around all sorts of 'passages' (crossroads, cemeteries, mills, bridges). They are forced to live separately and far away from the sanctified space inhabited by man and to keep their distance from things 'domesticated'. These forces must be chased away if ever they should come near and do harm to man. Incantations and exorcisms drive all suffering, sickness, hail and other evils 'up to the summits and into the mountains' or to the 'wild mountains and fruitless trees' or to the 'gorges' or even to 'the depths of the sea', 'forty fathoms deep in the earth'.

The intruding *stoicheia* , evil spirits (literally signifying 'elements'), are ostracized and banished, sent back where they belong, put back 'in their place'. Thus, the sacred inhabited space is well defined and safeguarded against any form of morbidity whether spiritual, physical or moral. On the other hand, since evil 'intrudes' and since people are able to chase it away, this means that they are also able to 'summon' it, and that is precisely what *mangania*, sorcery, and *vaskania*, 'casting the evil eye', do.

The cycle of human life and nature, the birth–death cycle, unfolds within a given and structured universe where time, space and species are not mixed, but are nonetheless connected by a series of symbolic relationships (analogical, metaphorical, metonymical, and so on). Thus, within this universe, animals, for instance, prognosticate what is in store for man, plants heal, mountains crack as a result of man's misfortunes, sexual intercourse impedes hunting, menstrual blood destroys plants, the weather is revealed by animal behaviour, holy water chases away evil spirits, specific periods of time have an influence on the transformation of beings and substances, the dead communicate with the living, saints mediate in the affairs of mortals, and human body fluids are influenced by external causes.

It is within this universe that the conception–birth–humanization process takes place, a process which assumes the dimensions of a cosmological drama. The centre of this dramatic stage is occupied by inhabited space, surrounded by the outer wild world, the underworld and the upper world (celestial world, heavens). However, it is a dynamic universe, in which both virtuous and malign powers, substances and beings, are in constant motion, thus influencing, forming, reinforcing or undermining man's destiny (Kyriakidan-Nestoros 1975:15–40; Stewart 1991:164–72).

Let us consider the plant fertility schema. In love songs the young woman is often signified by names of fruit trees or fruits – 'young apple tree' (*militsa*), 'young lemon tree' (*lemonitsa*), 'young bitter orange tree' (*nerantzoula*), 'orange', 'cherry' – or by aromatic flowers: 'rose', 'jasmin', 'myrtle':

> *'In the early morn she rose like a shrivelled apple*
> *like an apple, like a plum, like a cherry,*
> *to find her bodice untied and her lips touched by a kiss ...'*
> *'to take women young as apple trees and men young as cypresses...'* (Petropoulos 1954:33, 37, 39–47, Theros 1951, nos. 89, 101, 160, 166, 183, Frangaki 1969:78, 131, Politis 1914, Rodd 1892:266–8)

So that the lemon trees may be very fruitful, on returning from Easter Mass, the young daughter of the house would go over and kiss the lemon tree while uttering the following: 'Christ has risen, oh lemon tree, may the lemon tree bear as many lemons as there were people in the church' (Frangaki 1969: 131). And in the folk-story the childless woman keeps going to the river where the oleanders and myrtle trees grow and saying: 'if only I could have a little baby, even if the myrtle trees were to take it away from me', until finally she falls pregnant and gives birth to a baby girl (Loukatos 1957:72–5). In folk songs again, the daughter is often seen at a distance in the garden or the vineyard, and so the young man must find a way to approach her (Papazaphiropoulos 1887:123, 157; Kriaris 1909:167; Kalyvi 1938:11; Theros 1951:nos 40, 183; Petropoulos 1954:77; Papathanassi-Moussiopoulou 1981:49).

The wedding ceremony abounds with symbols of fertility and again they are fruits: apples, pomegranates, walnuts, hazelnuts, raisins. The standard held aloft in the wedding procession (which is also called 'apple' in Thrace) is made from tree branches to which a shred of fabric taken from the wedding-dress or a handkerchief was tied. Lemons, pomegranates, apples and occasionally other fruits were fixed to the ends of the branches. Sprays of ivy were placed in the bridal chamber, and people recited this verse: 'Just as ivy clings to the trees and spreads/may the bride be united with the bridegroom and take firm root', or they would sing: 'the blessed hour has arrived/for the carnation to be united with its golden clove' (Papamichael 1910:4; Saranti-Stamouli 1933:337; Megas 1939:128–9; Papathanassi-Maissiopoulou 1979:240). The symbolism of childbearing (especially when the child is male) is often very explicit. Form the lintel of the door was hung a wreath made from lemon tree branches with three lemons arranged in such a way so as to remind one of the male sexual organs. In other parts of Greece, once the bride sets out, the people sing: 'on the cord of the bridegroom's underpants/three pomegranates are hung/one a pomegranate, the other an apple/the third a fresh bunch of grapes'. (Romaios 1923:362)

A fairly widespread Greek wedding custom clearly illustrates the symbolic interrelation between the fertility of humans and the fertility of nature. As the bride enters her home she steps on the ploughshare, which has been placed on the threshold. This black bundle (which keeps evil away) locks within it a complete act of fertilization, from the beginning, i.e. cultivation – the ploughshare – to the end, i.e. the quintal, a balance used in the barn to weight wheat which is ready for consumption.[3] As another variation of the custom has it, before the bride enters her new home: 'straps are attached to her shoulder to which the bridegroom's oxen are tied, and in addition they put a plough in her hands'.

In Lefkada, childless women or women who wanted to give birth to a boy would step barefoot on two small ploughshares, kept in the church of St John. Once again, in a popular, well-known song with many versions, in reply to her complaining husband the childless mother says:

I gave you a field to sow and harvest
but if your oxen are meagre, your ploughs broken
and your ploughshare unwilling,
then what do you expect from me?'

In another version a young man, who has given up all the savings he made in a foreign land in order to spend the night with a Bulgarian girl, ends up falling asleep without doing anything and in the morning ask for the return of his fifteen hundred florins. The Bulgarian girl replies that:

> *I gave you a field to sow and harvest*
> *but if your oxen is sick, your plough broken*
> *and the ploughman a fumbler, who knows not how to plough . . .*
> *then off to the foreign land, oh stranger, go, and earn some more*. (Romaios 1923, Petropoulos 1954:77, Abbot 1903:176, Politis 1899–1902:280–1)

Among the means used for breaking a spell which has been cast over a couple, the so-called *ambodema* (tying), the following is mentioned: 'As he is ploughing the land, it sometimes happens that a ring gets tangled in the ploughshare. This ring the man passes round his genitals, and then has sexual intercourse.' (Dimitriou 1983:516)

The language used when referring to the subject of childbearing is also typical: the woman is reduced to her reproductive ability and is sometimes referred to as a *horafi*, i.e. 'field' ('he has a good field'). The words 'sow' and 'sowing' (*sperno*) are often used when referring to childbearing, the verb *genosperno* (a combination of the verb 'to give birth' and 'to sow' is used in an insulting way to refer to the couple's joint action in producing a child. The word *sporos*, 'seed', implies the sperm and the child – 'my father's seed', *tourkosporos*', 'seed of a Turkish man', *diavolosperma*, 'seed of the devil', while conception itself is expressed by the words *piano*, 'to catch', 'to take root', and *piasimo*, 'taken root', which also refer to the seeds of plants.[4]

With regard to questions little children ask in relation to how they came into the world, the typical answers they are given often refer to the world of plant life: 'I found you in a vineyard and took you home with me', 'I found you in a bed of nettles', 'you sprung from the ground like the grass and I took you home with me' (KL 1953 A:40; Lyberis 1975:138; Karapatakis 1979:94).

Moreover, the symbols of fertility found at wedding ceremonials also appears in other contexts, such as preparations for sowing time. The seeds are mixed with various fruits (walnuts, apples, almonds) and a small quantity of wheat from the previous year's harvest, while a pomegranate is placed inside the saddle-bag with the seeds to be eaten after the sowing is done.

Sometimes the pomegranate is cracked against the ploughshare (Loukopoulos 1938:180; Megas 1956:27).

The attitude according to which women are regarded as a field which is 'ploughed' by the man and is 'planted' with the male 'seed', rich in creative vitality and producing the 'fruit', goes back a long way in the Greek and wider Mediterranean region. Ancient Greek medicine, Judaso-Christian and Islamic traditions have been in constant dialogue for centuries. They have formed many of the conceptions which rule both intellectual and folk ways of thinking in the civilizations in the region (Cf. Musallam 1983; Gelis 1984; Delaney 1986,1990; du Bois 1988; but also Dube 1986; Brandstrom 1990).

The types of food that are forbidden during pregnancy are few in number, and mainly concern food obtained from wild plants and animals with a particular symbolic content or with traits that are recognized as being disgusting from a physical or moral point of view. Therefore, the consumption of hare is prohibited – a dietary taboo particularly widespread in Europe and the East. If hare is eaten by the mother, the newly-born child will be unable to sleep properly, sleeping only lightly, or (rarely mentioned) the child with be born with a fissure of the upper lip, i.e. it will suffer from harelip. The hare is generally considered an unlucky animal, since it leaves its young very soon, a belief which is reflected in proverbs: 'the hare's little ones have scattered', and 'do not resemble the hare, that bears its young and then denies them'. The hare is a symbol of cowardice, the devil and fertility. In fact, it is believed to change sex from time to time. (KL 2125:20; KL 2135:8; KL 1566:9; KL 1424:21; KL 1405:1; KL 1845:3; KL 2143:44; KL 1674:2; Politis 1904: nos 182, 841, 849).

The consumption of snails is prohibited during pregnancy because the child will become *saliariko*, that is a 'driveller', or *kahektio*, i.e. sickly' (Cf. Musallam 1983; Gélis 1984; Delaney 1986,1991; du Bois 1988; but also Psychogios 1951:346; Frangaki 1978:36; Dube 1986; Brandstrom 1990). In this case also, we are dealing with 'wild' food, which, by its ability to come out of its shell but retreat into it again, reminds us of the image of a foetus which starts coming down the birth canal but threatens to go back into its mother's womb.

False pregnancy, or *anemogastri*/*anemogastria* as it is called, literally 'being pregnant from the air', is considered the devil's doing. The *anemos* or *aeras* i.e. 'wind', refers to the devil or some kind of evil spirit or demon. This is euphemistically implied by the expressions *aei ston anemo*, i.e. 'go off with the wind', *pai ston anemo*, i.e. 'he/she is gone off with the wind', and the names of cunning spirits called *anemikes*, *aeroudes* and *anemogazoudes*, which are related to certain physical or mental illnesses (*anembodisma*, 'wind-impediment') which threaten or have an effect mainly on those who are in a liminal state – newly-born, women in labour, pregnant women, 'newly-weds (Lambrakis 1915:107; Kyriakidis 1922:189–203; Politis 1931:51–63). According to a tradition belonging to Thrace, God cursed the devil, saying to him, 'dwell in the wind and remain up there until you rot', and the devil went off to the heavens from where he conducts his evil doings. Thus, false pregnancy is generally considered the devil's doing, taking advantage of 'the woman's strong desire', or an undertaking of a bad spirit, 'a fairy who makes a vvv... sound at night' (KL 2125:19; KL 1699:34; KL 1566:3; Megas 1929:390; Chowmouziadis 1940:70–1; Konsolas 1966:229. Cf. Ephesians 2:2;6:12).

In some areas false pregnancy is considered the consequence of wind entering the womb and inflating it – *anemofouskoma*, 'swelling by the wind' (Limnos) or *anemopordos*, 'crepitus ventris of the wind' (Lesvos), since the child is not really a child at all but a 'fart' – which is something that could happen when a woman is defecating in the countryside, therefore far away from her familiar places, in the open or in the wilderness (Crete). However, the prevailing idea in those parts is that the devil is able to penetrate the abdomen of a human body 'like the wind' (KL 1844 A:1; KL 1631:3; Frangaki 1978:40, 164; Karapatakis 1979:30). Again wilderness is related to some kind of non-legitimate sexuality. False pregnancy may, however, serve as an excuse for those women who get rid of their child, either because it is *klefto*, i.e. 'clandestine', 'illegitimate', or because they are up to their eyes in children and have already got one too many (Psychogios 1951:342).

BREADMAKING

In most part of Greece, priests did not accept the *prosphoron*, the bread for the Eucharist, prepared by a sterile or infertile woman, often called *alitourgiti* (a person who has not received communion). The only exception was on the name day of the childless couple when the priest himself brought the Holy Bread to the couple's house (KL 2143:41; KL 1653:11; Vanazounta 1963:522; Konsolas 1966:228; Regas 1980:49). In Sciathos the married couple abstained from Holy Communion until they had their first child (Regas 1970;49). The reason according to the priests was that bread 'resembles Christ that the Virgin took over to the church' or as the Church officially states in the *Pedalion* (the Canon Law of the Orthodox Church), the bread is consecrated because it was offered to God and because 'it stands for a model [*typos*, 'type'] of Theotokos' [Mother of God's] belly'. The quotation continues: 'Just as the Lamb of God came out from her body, so from the oblation comes out the Lamb to be mystically officiated' and later on, 'the Holy Bread signifies [*semainei*] Theotokos' belly' (Pedalion: 408 n. 1, 681–3 n. 3). It is interesting that the refusal by the Church to accept bread also applies in the case of prostitutes and concubines, that is women who are 'attracted by pleasure', who give themselves to 'carnal love', thus remaining at odds with fertility and the possibility of becoming a mother (Pedalion: 19, 683). The Holy Bread and any other oblation have to be made exclusively from wheat, 'for the Lord likened his holy Body to wheat' (Pedalion: 682).

But this refusal has its profane equivalent: a childless woman never plants a field for fear 'that the wheat also will become barren'. And no one takes yeast from a childless woman to make bread. Interestingly enough, the yeast for leavening bread is often called *manna* (mother) (KL 1675:1; Salvanos 1929:146; Vanazounta 1963:522; Kensolas 1966:228; Karapatakis 1978:8). In Crete it was believed that a woman leaving too many crumbs of bread on the table will have many children.

A ritual against sterility uses the metaphor of bread-making, combining the sacred and profane aspects of bread. When a new watermill is built 'women make the barren woman seat on the millstone and let her revolve until a small quantity of wheat has been ground. This flour is then used to knead the bread that she sends to the priest, and after consecrating it he conducts a divine service in her name.' Here the whole transformation of the seeds (nature) to flour then to dough then again to bread, which *fouskoni*, 'swells in the oven' (culture), symbolically repeats the act of procreation, which is metonymically related on the one hand to the sacred and on the other to the sterile person. One of the names given to a pregnant woman is *fouskomeni*, that is 'swollen'.

On the other hand, a plant called *stirouvotano* or *atechnohorto* (i.e. 'sterility herb' or 'childlessness herb') believed to cause sterility for seven years and used for preventing conception, is considered so powerful that it can stop the millstone of the water-mill, even if only a tiny piece of the herb comes in contact with it. The same logic pertains to the custom followed by the barren woman of eating bread from a new oven: in a symbolic inversion the product of the oven's 'fertility' is inserted into the mouth of the barren woman to be delivered from her womb as a product of human fertility (KL 1566:1; Athanassopoulos 1915:408–9; Megas 1939:121; Frangaki 1978:31).

WEAVING

One of the most widely spread divinatory means of foretelling the sex of the future child is connected with the loom, a dominant symbol of womanhood in Greek culture as in other Mediterranean and Middle Eastern cultures (Bourdieu 1970; Servier 1985:242–3). When a piece of woven material is completed and the woman unwind it from the cloth beam (*anti*), they let fall or take out the *vergha* or *gardio*, i.e. the rod that fits on the groove of the cloth beam and holds the woven material or web. A woman holds the rod in her teeth and 'having in mind' (*meletái*) the pregnant woman she comes out the house with her eyes closed. (The verb *meletáo* in this context also means to 'mention the name of someone or something', to 'think about', to 'read up'). If the first person the woman sees passing by when she opens her eyes is a woman, the child will be born a girl; if it is a man, it will be a boy (KL 1405:2; KL 1566:3; KL 1631:5; KL 2125:20; Keramida 1932:452; Sanders 1962:129; Marinellis 1978:180; Karapatakis 1979:32; Handman 1980:185).

The whole process of weaving is a particularly symbolically charged process where two (taxonomically) discrete principles or categories like the vertical and horizontal, the passive and active (the warp and the weft), the female and the male come in contact. Weaving is metaphorically equated to pregnancy, while the rod which is inside the roll of woven material – in its 'belly' as it were – comes out (is born) with the completion of the weaving process and is related metonymically to the pregnant woman. Sometimes the pregnant woman herself holds the rod in her teeth. In another variation of this prognostication the women throw behind their backs in the street the *xetrachiloma*, i.e. the small, round piece that they remove from the woven cloth when making a new night-dress in order to pass it over the head and neck of the woman. Then they wait to ascertain the sex of the first person passing by. Here too we have a symbolic inversion of down and front to up and behind.

But this particular meaning of weaving comes out in other contexts as well. When a woman begins to weave a new piece of cloth she wishes: 'may the good time come and an easy unweaving' (*i ora i kali ki kali ksifasi*); 'unweaving' here means completion of the weaving rather than 'unstitch' or 'unsew', and 'good time' is opposed to 'bad time' – *kakïa ora*, the 'dangerous hour' (see, e.g. Blum and Blum 1970). The same wishes are addressed to the pregnant woman: 'may the good time come and have an easy liberation' (*i ora i kali kai lefteria*). Again the front part of the warp, which is attached to the beam and is not woven (about a span long called *decadologia*), is hung on infertile trees in order to make them bear fruits. On the other hand the last part of the warp (which also is not woven) is hung on the loom which must always be full and never empty.

The web itself, the completed piece of woven material, is sometimes 'twice churched', literally, 'twice forty days' (*diplosarantisma*), which means it has taken more than eighty days to be completed. In this case the rod of the cloth beam has a special power to foretell the sex of the coming child. This obviously refers to the forty days' seclusion of the mother and her newborn child, until churching, when both are purified and incorporated into the community.

The pregnant woman has also to refrain from touching the warp or weft of the loom during pregnancy, lest the umbilical cord gets coiled around the child's neck (Konsolas 1966:233; Marinellis 1978:179; Karapatakis 1979:28–9). The first half metre of the woven material, called *kombodessi*, i.e. 'tied knots', is never used for making a male shirt or trousers, otherwise the man wearing them will be 'tied down' (*denetai*), i.e. will become impotent. On the other side the *kombodessi* or *kombodetires* are tied to the pregnant woman's underwear to protect her from aborting (KL 2125:19; Regas 1970:318; Frangaki 1974: 42–7). Furthermore, the woman weaving must not leave the *korfo*, the area between the cloth beam and the reed holding the warp threads, empty at night, that is, she must complete this unwoven part, otherwise temptation comes at night and starts weaving (the loom must not be left 'open'). The process of weaving is also connected to the Moirai, the Fates who carry a spindle and yarn and spin every child's thread of life and destiny.[5] This is perhaps why the weaving metaphor is so often related to prognostication. The Fates in a way speak through the loom.

But weaving is also related to the moon that is continuously waxing and waning. The books of Solomon, and older treatises on magic, portray the moon as a woman holding a distaff and spinning (Politis [1921]1975:185; also du Boulay 1991:57). Sometimes the moon is conceived as a cow that could be brought to earth to be milked for the purposes of love magic. Everywhere in Greece the moon is related to images of fertility, renewal, creativity as that of the weaver, of the lactiferous cow, of gestation, of fertile and generative influence on plants, animals, marriages, births, affairs and health matters. People plant and sow during the waxing of the moon (*ghémosi* – the 'filling of the moon') 'so that the seeds will grow in the fields or in the belly of one's wife. One does not plant in the moon's waning for the seeds in the field will fail and one's wife will be barren.' On the whole the waning of the moon increases all kinds of dangers and misfortunes (KL 1566:17; KL 1628:5, Politis 1874:216, [1921]1975:184–211; Vanazounta 1964:522,524; Blum and Blum 1965:31: Karapatakis 1979:32; du Boulay 1991:57–60; cf. Opie and Tatem 1989:261–4 for similar beliefs in Anglo-Saxon cultures).

CONCLUSION

I take a constructivist position on metaphor, maintaining that the objective world is not transparent and directly accessible but is constructed culturally by people living in particular social and historical settings. And metaphors in this tradition are instrumental in creating reality, they are cognitive instruments. In this sense I am closer to those who argue that metaphor is a form of thought (Sapir and Crocker 1977; Lakoff and Johnson 1980; Holland and Quinn 1987; MacCormack 1990).

Metaphors are part of what people use to interpret the world and act on it. In this sense they underlie all kinds of theories, cultural, scientific, religious or whatever. The questions posed by every discipline, including our, derive from the metaphors that drive these theories. Let us remember the different metaphoric conceptions of society in our discipline. We have started with the idea of society as biological organism, moved to the idea of society as machine, then a language, as text, as dialogue, as melodic or cacophonic co-existence of different discourses (Brown 1977:ch.4; Salmond 1982; Parkin 1987:53–4). Remember the sometimes 'Byzantine' debates over the base, structure and superstructure in Marxist spatial metaphor. If this applies to learned theories it must certainly also apply to folk theories (Salmond 1982; see also Sternberg 1990 who examines several metaphors that underlie theories of intelligence).

But metaphor in its limited sense (as the device which establishes a relation of similarity between two unlike domains or things and thus a relation of equivalence) is only one of various kinds of metaphoric modes of thought, or tropes. Metonymy (the establishment of a relation of conceptual, spatial or temporal contiguity), synecdoche, homology, analogy, translation, opposition, contradiction, are all important aspects of the metaphoric mechanisms with which people create their worlds.[6] In the case of the metaphors here presented, the seed/earth metaphor for example, what I have tried to do is show that it is not an isolated kind of trope. Such a view would lead to a microscopic approach that would study individual sentence-level metaphors, independently of others. The material here suggests that the seed/earth metaphor is much more extended, making use of the many aspects of vegetative life, and relating at the same time to other kinds of metaphors.

What I was able to find in the metaphors I have presented here, but also in other metaphors (and in ritual practices which encompass metaphoric thinking) is an underlying cultural schema that connects different domains of the world. In the case of the seed/earth metaphor a cultural scheme emerges that is based on the idea of a distinction between, on the one hand, sexuality, sensuality, embodiment and nature, and on the other (a-sexual) motherhood, morality, spirituality, culture.[7] This is a distinction which we find again in the Eve/Virgin Mary dichotomy, or between biological birth and baptism (second birth) (cf. Bloch and Guggenheim 1981) in both ecclesiastical and folk contexts.

In Greece, Campbell and others have argued that social identity is very closely linked to gender. This approach focuses on the household, the family and marriage. Identity is defined at the meeting point of the two sexes. Identity is thus considered as something already biologically given. The elements that constitute identity have been allocated, as it were, to men and women. In the domestic division of labour, gender and identity are in a close complementary relation. Identity is contained in the roles, in the properties of action. This is a reduction of the scope of identity, in that we are principally and in essence talking about gender and married procreative heterosexuality. We are also limited by the fact that we are talking about man and woman from the point if view of roles, of the normative patterns, of the functions that they must perform: what I am and what I do are aspects of an ordered reality, of a normative pattern: I do what I have to do.

By exploring the different aspects – metaphoric, metonymic, linguistic or ritual – of procreation (both here and in other research) I have been able to refer to a wider and more open version of identity, able, that is, to refer not to role and function, but to an ontology, to the folk ontology, the 'little tradition' which I relate then to the ecclesiastical and other traditions. (Juliet du Boulay is most certainly working in a similar direction). This ontology was constituted by approaching the whole issue processually, by taking into account the sequence of ritual practices unfolding processually in time, and among other things by exploring the general cultural schemas or models that underlie metaphors pertaining to different domains of people's life in addition to birth and procreation, like death, marriage, baptism.

As a result I have ended up in my wider research examining substances (blood, sperm, saliva, milk), influences (natural, supernatural, demonic, astral), folk theories, social reality, cosmic reality, ritual attitudes, divinatory practices, and properties that allow each individual, male or female, to be distinguished from fellow humans.

NOTES

*I would like to thank Peter Loizos for his comments and encouragement, and Alexandra Bakalaki for her help to me in writing this paper.

1 A large part of the material comes in the form of manuscripts from the archives of the Center for Research on Greek Folklore in Athens. References to these archives include, after the abreviation KL, the manuscript and page number.

2 For a discussion of folklore in Greece, see Herzfeld 1982.

3 The same logic pertains to the custom of putting a *stateri* (quintal) – symbol of the completion of an act – near a dying person in order to help his or her soul to depart peacefully (Romaios 1923:353).

4 MLEG s.v. *'chorafi'* (field), *'sperno'* (to plant), *'sporos'* (seed), *'arotro'* (plough) ILLA s.v. *'gennosperma'*, Tsitselis 1874:186–7. The greek verb *aro* (to plough) meant to copulate, the word *arotron* (plough) in the plural, *arotra*, meant genitals, the word *aroura* (field for ploughing and sowing) meant also vagina and the word *arotos* (ploughing) procreation. Cf. the Sanskrit langala (plough) and *langula* (penis).

5 The theme is amply documented, as nearly all sources refer to this connection. See also Abbott 1903:126–9, Campbell 1964:329–31, du Boulay 1974:82, Blum and Blum 1970:100.

6 J. Overing (1991:158 quoting Searle 1979) stresses the 'importance of background factual information for their comprehension, we must share with the speaker the relevant understanding.and knowledge about the world'.

7 On the opposition between sexuality and fertility see Bloch and Parry 1982. Cf also Pina-Cabral 1986:99–100, 104–9.

CHAPTER 11

PROCREATION, PATRIARCHY AND MEDICAL SCIENCE

RESISTANCE TO RECOGNIZING MATERNAL CONTRIBUTIONS IN EUROPEAN EMBRYOLOGICAL THOUGHT

JULIA STONEHOUSE

The facts of human reproduction were extremely difficult to establish scientifically, taking 133 years from inception of the correct theory – in 1827 with the discovery of the mammalian ovum – to actual proof in 1960 – when photomicrographs of ovum and sperm fusing, and subsequent cell division, were observed as part of *in vitro* fertilization (IVF) experimentation.[1] This long road to discovery was not a case of filling in the detailed mechanics of something we basically knew – in simple terms, that there are two parents with generative 'seed' and the fusion of that 'seed'; but of disproving what we thought we knew – there is one 'seed', and it is male.

There was no one piece of the experimental jigsaw that categorically proved the facts of life, although the theory was tight enough by 1900 for most sceptics to be intellectually fought off. However, because the experimental work was being done on frogs, sea urchins, fruit flies and garden peas, those people who believed there is a fundamental difference between humans and other life forms took longer to convince.

The details of reproduction were revealed by generations of embryologists who, collectively, did for the study of life what Kepler had done for astronomy and Galileo for physics.[2] Key players were Antoni van Leeuwenhoek, Karl Ernst von Baer, Oskar Hertwig and Hermann Fol. Yet these people remain unknown to the general public, and the whole subject of the discovery of the facts of life has been relegated to the shelves of specialist medical libraries, for reasons discussed later in this article.

Meanwhile, it is common to read in history books that 'men discovered their role in reproduction around 8000 BC' – although men and women discovered their true role in reproduction almost 10,000 years later. The 8000 BC date is significant to archaeologists because that is when the phallus and intercourse first make an appearance in artefact. Prior to this, people created many images of vulvas, breasts and protruding abdomens – signs of female generativity – so it is thought people then believed women produced babies parthenogenetically, without men. This may have been conceptualized as 'you pluck a baby from the woman, as you pluck a fruit from a tree, or a root from the ground'. After 8000 BC, the likelihood is that men were perceived as waterers – the source of irrigation crucial to make the seed, already in the woman, germinate and grow – much as perennial seeds in the ground respond to rainfall. The evidence for this comes from early inheritance law, mythology, linguistics and artefact. There came a point, however, roughly 3000 BC, when ideas began to change again, with the male being seen as the source of human seed, which he planted in the soil of the woman – now perceived as an incubator and not a generant as such. This later theory, in all its many aspects, is the subject of this article.

There proved to be many ways of presenting the argument that life is transmitted through males only. Along with the simple observation 'no ram = no lamb', the idea that man's seed is planted in the nutritive but non-generative soil of the woman was common. Chickens could be seen to produce eggs without there being a cockerel, but live chicks failed to appear. In humans, Aristotle thought in terms of generative male semen mixing with non-generative menstrual blood while Galen, who thought female sexual secretions were a 'seed' which came from the ovaries, said it 'contributes nothing to the generation of offspring', 'because she is colder' – an argument he 'proved' by drawing the abdominal veins incorrectly, as we shall see.

In these theories, the essential spark of life was seen to be conveyed in male semen, to the womb, where it was nurtured and otherwise influenced by material contributed by the female body. Embryological debate largely centred on which female materials were involved, such as menstrual blood, sexual secretions, the ovaries, womb, amniotic fluid, placenta or umbilical cord.

The question of life affected past ancestry, control over progeny, a person's relationship to God, especially with regard to creativity and spirituality, and, of course, inheritance. In 1776, half a century before the discovery of the mammalian ovum, the writer James Boswell had to decide whether to leave his estate to heirs of both sexes, or to male heirs only. He wrote:

> I had a zealous partiality for heirs male, however remote, which I maintained by arguments which appeared to me to have considerable weight. As, first, the opinion of some distinguished naturalists, that our species is transmitted through males only, the female being all along no more than a nidus, or nurse, as Mother Earth is to plants of every sort; which notion seems to be confirmed by that of scripture – 'He was yet in the loins of his Father when Melchizedek met him' (Heb. v11.10).
>
> (Boswell 1776:II 428)

The idea that 'our species is transmitted through males only' was the predominant view in Europe and the Middle East, until around the turn of the twentieth century. It is salutary then, when looking at cultures with theories different to our own contemporary view, to remember our own recent ignorance, which very negatively influenced the position of women in both law and social culture.

Deeply held beliefs about procreation are aspects of spirituality, and to challenge them is to challenge 'nature' and the commonly believed source of nature, which many call 'God'. At the same time, incorrect biological 'facts' of life can be extrapolated from, and conclusions drawn about, the fundamental 'nature' of men and women, as can be seen throughout the written history of embryology.

THE ANCIENT GREEKS

In Athens, as elsewhere in Europe and the Middle East, male kinship was preceded by female kinship (Frazer [1890]1980: 155). The transition was to take many centuries. In 458 BC, Athens saw the first performance of Aeschylus' drama *Eumenides*, in which Apollo successfully defends Orestes from the charge of murdering his mother, using the argument that there can be no charge of matricide because there is no such thing as a 'mother':

> The mother is not the true source of life,
> We call her mother, but she is more the nurse,
> The furrow where the seed is thrust.
> The thruster, the father, is the true parent:
> The woman but tends the growing plant
> With god's good grace, the host
> That shelters the stranger-guest.'
> (Aeschylus 1953:114)

The casting vote was the goddess Athene's, who in pre-Hellenic times was said to have emerged from the womb of lake Tritonis, but who by this time, significantly, was said to have been born from the head of her father, Zeus's, after he had swallowed her mother, Metis. With this drama-propaganda, the audience were entreated to accept the new reproductive theory, as Athene had apparently done.

The philosopher Plato (427–347 BC) was convinced, writing in *The Republic* that the male and female sex 'differ only in just this respect that the female bears and the male begets' (Plato 1982:5.5, p. 445). His pupil, Aristotle, was likewise persuaded. But there were still those prepared to argue for a female contribution to generation, including the older Hippocrates (460–370 BC) and, as late as 320 BC, the fundamentally equalist Epicurius, who argued a doctrine of two seeds – which competed for some centuries with the Aristotelean theory of a sole male generant. But as the old notion of a female seed faded with time, the whole concept of two seeds became increasingly difficult to accept. After all, we plant singular seeds in the nutritive ground, from which singular plants grow.

The most enduring influences on European and Middle Eastern thought were Artistotle and Galen. They had different theories, but neither thought the female was generative.

Aristotle

Aristotle (384–322 BC) knew of a female fish, 'erythrinus',[3] which reproduced parthenogenetically, on its own, and concluded, because 'nature does nothing in vain', in those animals with two genders it must be the male that 'always completes the business of generation'. He noted that 'semen begins to appear in males and to be emitted at the same time of life that the menstrual flow begins', and that 'in the decline of life the generative power fails in the one sex and the menstrual discharge in the other' (Aristotle 1984:II i, 727.a.5–10). From this, Aristotle deduced that menstruation 'is analogous in females to the semen in males', ignoring the fact that one is related to the calendar and the other to sex, but using this logic; 'It is plain that the female does not contribute semen to the generation of the offspring. For if she had semen she would not have menstrual fluid; but as it is, because she has the latter she has not the former' (ibid.: a. 27–30). He concluded that woman's 'prime matter' was given 'form' by the male seed.

Aristotle believed that both menstrual blood and semen derived from blood, but that the blood in women received insufficient heat to concoct semen. Men's blood, having enough heat, did produce generative semen – white and of little quantity; but women's blood couldn't boil to perfection, as it were, and remained red and profuse. Women were described as imperfect men, like underdeveloped, pre-adolescent boys.

Aristotle said men delivered the 'impetus and form' (the energy and blueprint for a new life), as well as 'the sentient soul; (the thinking, creative part), while women contributed the 'matter'. He used different analogies to describe the transformative role of men, including the widespread 'milk and rennet' theory, writing, 'The male emits semen into the female and upon entry of the semen the young animals are "set" and constituted and assume their proper shape.' He put it another way: 'the male semen cooks and shapes menstrual blood into a new human being'.

He also said men were like carpenters who, with their creative force, make an object, a baby, using the material of the woman, the wood. On the basis of his biology, Aristotle concluded that, 'The male stands for the effective and the active, and the female ... for the passive', noting elsewhere, 'of course the active elements are always higher on any scale, and more divine' (Aristotle 1984:II i, 732.a.3–10). This led him to advocate segregation: 'as the first efficient or moving cause, to which belong the definition and the form, is better and more divine in its nature than the material on which it works, it is better that the superior principle should be separated from the inferior. Therefore, whenever it is possible and so far as it is possible, the male is separated from the female' (ibid.). It did not stop there: 'the relation of the male to the female is naturally that of the superior to the inferior – of the ruling to the ruled' (Politics, I v,1254b, 12–16). Aristotle also said that women's 'minds, unlike their bodies, should be kept free from exertion', because 'children evidently draw on the mother who carries them in her womb, just as plants draw on the soil'.

Aristotle did at least endow women with souls, unlike many who came after, although he said woman's imperfect body precluded her from being able to pass soul onto the children.

Galen

Galen of Pergamos (AD 129–199), often called 'the founder of experimental physiology', thought women produced a 'seed' that came from the ovaries (said to have been discovered around 300 BC by the Greek anatomist, Herophilus, but certainly known of before that). Galen identified this seed with female sexual secretions of which he wrote: 'this liquid not only stimulates to the sexual act but also gives pleasure and moistens the passageway as it escapes'. Elsewhere, he wrote that it gives nourishment, and this was the aspect of Galen's theory emphasized in later, more puritanical times. Contrary to Aristotle, Galen was prepared to accept the female 'seed' contributed 'a source of movement', but he was clear as to it's role in reproduction, writing that it 'contributes nothing to the generation of offspring', the reason given being 'because she is colder' (Galen 1968:14.11.295).

Galen was working with three theories which were common at the time, including the idea that bodily fluids derive from blood. He also believed the 600-year-old theory of Empedocles, that the 'hot' elements of fire and air are essentially male while the 'cold' elements of earth and water are essentially female' and the Hippocratic idea that female children are created by combining the 'seed' from the left ovary with seed from the left testicle, with the resultant combination developing on the left side of the uterus. Galen wrote, 'the female must have smaller, less perfect testes, and the semen generated in them must be scantier, colder and wetter (for these things too follow of necessity from the deficient heat)' (Galen 1968:14.11.301).

The reason for this supposed lack of heat on the left side of the body needed to be explained, and Galen did it with some 'very creative anatomy', as biology historian Nancy Tuana puts it (Tuana 1989a:156). Galen incorrectly drew the abdominal veins supplying organs on the left side, showing them bypassing the kidneys, unlike those on the right. He wrote: 'the left testis in the male and the left uterus in the female received blood still uncleansed, full of residues, watery and serous'. According to Galen, as the blood going to the left side is impure, it contains less heat, and cannot perform well enough to facilitate the development of perfect, i.e. generative, seed.

Galen saw a similarity in shape between the penis/testicles and the vagina/womb/ovaries (Galen 1968:14.11.297), and attributed this to the female lack of heat, saying a woman's genitals 'were formed within her when she was still a foetus, but could not because of the defect in the heat emerge and project on the outside' (ibid.: 14.11.299). They had not 'popped-out', so to speak, and proved that woman were underdeveloped men, unable to reproduce.

JUDAISM, CHRISTIANITY AND ISLAM

The Levite priests who bought Judaism to Canaan four thousand years ago had a very hard time convincing the locals to give up worshipping 'the Queen of Heaven', and using idols – the images of their goddess Astarte. Indeed, the Old Testament can be read from Adam and Eve to the last words of Malachi[4] as the story of the battle between the older matriarchal system and the new patriarchal one.

The 'milk and rennet' concept of reproduction, also elucidated by Aristotle amongst others, is here described in the Jewish Midrash Rabbah 14, 19:

> A mother's womb is full of standing blood, which flows therefrom in menstruation. But, at God's will, a drop of whiteness enters and falls into its midst and behold a child is formed. This is likened unto a bowl of milk; when a drop of rennet falls into it, it congeals and stands; if not it continues as liquid.

Although the essential spark of life is here conferred by the male, the Jewish line has always descended through the female line. This paradox may be explained by the ancient nature of this religion and by the early women's reluctance to surrender parental rights. Perhaps a concession was made, at an early date, and just continued as tradition despite the male-centred view of life, which got stronger as time went on. The more usual explanation is that, as the woman is the centre of the home, children will be brought up Jewish even if the father is absent, or the child is the result of infidelity with a gentile man.

In the Bible, Genesis 2:7, it is said: 'The Lord God formed man of the dust of the ground and breathed into his nostrils the breath of life; and man became a living soul.' At no point did God breathe into the nostrils of woman 'the breath of life' which, from a reproduction theory point of view, can be interpreted as generative capacity. Certainly, when talking about lineage and 'seed', the Bible refers only to men. In Genesis 5 it was Adam who 'begat a son in his own likeness, after his image' and Seth who 'begat sons and daughters'. Genesis 6:1 states that 'men began to multiply on the face of the earth, and daughters were born unto them', while in Genesis 12:7 'the Lord appeared unto Abram, and said, Unto they seed will I give this land'.

In Luke 3:23–38, the genealogy of Jesus starts with Joseph, who was the son of Heli, the son of Matthat, the son of Levi, the son of Melchi, the son of Janna, the son of Joseph, etc., and goes all the way back through a total of 75 generations of men, to Adam. In Corinthians 11:7–9 we are told that man should not cover his head in church because 'he is in the image and glory of God: but the woman is the glory of the man; For the man is not of the woman; but the woman of the man.'

In the Quran, Sura 2:223 it is written: 'Women are given to you as fields to be sown, so go to them and sow [your seed] as you wish.' The Islamic scholar Raghib wrote in *Safinat*:

> Learned men declare that sperm, when placed in the uterus, is first transformed into a small, round ball, while keeping its original white colour. And this lasts for six days. At the centre of this ball then appears a spot of blood. This spot will be the confluence of the souls [*multaqa al arwah*]. When the creation is completed this will be the heart.[5]

There is only sperm and uterus, no ovum or female seed for the sperm to meet and fuse with. This reflects the Quranic facts of human creation by God, which is framed in terms of 'a drop', in 'a receptacle secure':

> We created man of an extraction of clay,
> then We set him, a drop, in a receptacle secure,
> then We created of the drop a clot
> then We created of the clot a tissue
> then We created of the tissue bones
> then We garmented the bones in flesh;
> thereafter we produced him as another creature.
> So blessed be God, the fairest of creators!

It was difficult in any Christian or Islamic area to challenge the *status quo* – a masculinist reproduction theory. It could be called blasphemy.

FROM THE GREEKS TO THE SIXTEENTH-CENTURY

Partly due to Church prohibition of anatomical dissection in Europe, Galen's anatomy was to stand for over 1,500 years. Flemish anatomist Andreas Vesalius (1514–64) discovered the fiction of the abdominal veins, but he chose to ignore this and to perpetuate Galen's 'facts' (perhaps because he was in enough theological trouble for not being able to confirm Adam's missing rib and the heart bone of biblical reference). Ambrose Pare (1517–90) was another who propagated Galen's ideas, drawing the womb and vagina as undescended testicles and penis – supposedly underdeveloped and thus incapable of generation.

Men of learning made pronouncements glorifying the male contribution and denigrating the female element, along with the female herself. Medical schools in Europe taught that women had 'semen', but declared it was 'ignoble', lacking in 'copious spirit', or 'useless and vitiated' – i.e. imperfect or faulty. By comparison, male semen was attributed with the crucial reproductive powers. The twelfth-century anatomist Ricardo Anglici said sperm (by which he meant semen) provides the 'spirit and creative power and form', while Thomas Aquinas in the thirteenth century declared that men's 'active seminal power' gives form to the 'corporeal matter, which is supplied by the mother'. The thirteenth-century scholar Giles of Rome believed that a woman 'consists of a slippery and fluid *materia* which can only retain the impress of the form in the womb when it is in the presence of the agent, the male semen'. He extrapolated from this notion, saying women had a cold, moist and slippery nature and were, therefore, unstable and untrustworthy (Atkinson 1991:51).

Leonardo da Vinci knew an Italian married to an Ethiopian, and their children, and said, around 1500, 'the seed of the female was as potent as that of the male in generation' (quoted in Needham 1934:80). Nobody took much notice though and Leonardo, seeking less controversial subjects perhaps, turned his attention to the design of flying machines and submarines.

THE SEVENTEENTH AND EIGHTEENTH CENTURIES

Radical change in thinking came about after two crucial discoveries in the Dutch city of Delft. In 1672 a young surgeon, Reinier de Graaf, discovered in a rabbit what he thought was an ovum, but what we now know to be the Graafian follicle – the sac which encases an ovum. However, as the ovary and whatever it contained had for so long been thought of as nutritive, this new 'ovum' was generally seen as an item of nutritive material, a loaf in a basket, food for the growing baby within. Nevertheless, it subsequently became an important new component in the debate.

Meanwhile, a Delft cloth merchant, Antoni van Leeuwenhoek was making microscopes to examine thread. He subsequently used them to discover blood cells, bacteria in plaque from teeth, and small creatures living in drops of water taken from ponds, and in time became known as 'the father of microbiology and protozoology'. Embryological history was changed, however, in 1675, when Leeuwenhoek looked at semen, and saw sperm.

In his role as a correspondent of the Royal Society in London, de Graaf introduced Leeuwenhoek's amateur work to the world of academic science. Writing of the discovery some 178 years later, in 1853, the German zoologist Leuckart said: 'there is scarcely any discovery in the realm of animal biology which has aroused so general an interest as the discovery of these motile seminal corpuscles'. Leeuwenhoek thought each sperm contained the whole body of the child, as an insect larva is an earlier stage of the insect it becomes. Others thought in terms of miniature people, an unfolding of something preformed.

As it transpired, microscopes with the same extraordinary power of magnification could not be replicated for 150 years.

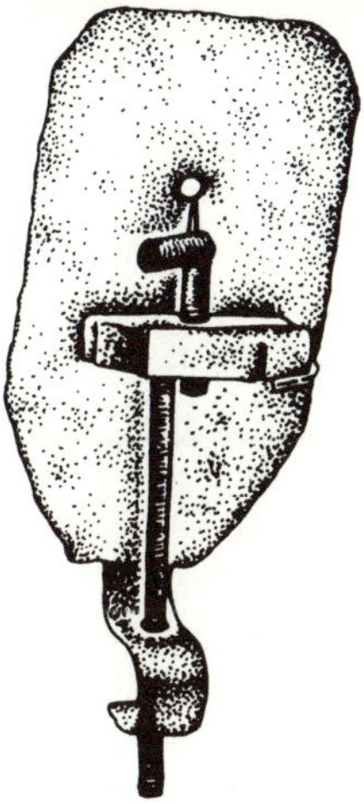

In 1675 Leeuwenhoek discovered sperm by looking at semen placed in a very small glass tube affixed to the spike facing the 3 mm lens, which was incorporated into a piece of flat, beaten brass. The total height of the microscope was 7 cm, and positioning of the spike was accomplished by means of the two vertical screws.

This was a great pity as Leeuwenhoek wouldn't hire, lend or sell any of his fantastic microscopes during his lifetime and although they were sold at auction on his death, they all strangely disappeared. Other researchers could not therefore replicate his work, or take the examination of the Graafian follicle further.

Epigenesis and pre-formation

Throughout embryological history, the fundamental question was whether the baby is a new creation formed from both male and female material, or an unfolding, preformed seed – the theories of epigenesis and preformation respectively. 'Epigenesis' may convey the idea of equality, but Aristotle and Galen were both epigenesists and neither propounded generative equality.

As a theory, epigenesis was stopped in its tracks by the two discoveries in Delft. Science decamped to an either/or position: either the baby was preformed in the sperm, or in the so-called 'ovum'. 'Preformation doctrine', as it became known, held that the 'seed' (be that sperm or 'ovum') contains a potential person which (if male or female respectively) carries future generations of seed within them. In other words, all human life was encapsulated at the beginning of time in the body of either Adam or Eve.

The ovist position was, of course, highly contentious as it challenged the order of things as told in Genesis 2:23: God fashioned Eve from one of Adam's ribs and Adam said, 'This is now bone of my bone, flesh of my flesh; and shall be called woman, because she was taken out of man.' Ovism implied that, on the contrary, woman did not come from man, but man from woman.

There were good arguments against preformation doctrine in general. Caterpillars metamorphose into butterflies and lizards can grow new tails, birds new feathers and crustacea new claws. If they had been preformed at creation, they wouldn't be able to 'create' anew. In 1683 Brunner argued against preformation doctrine by saying that if, as was generally believed, monsters were the direct result of the mental state of pregnant women, the child could not have been preformed at creation.

The strongest argument against preformation was the sheer numbers involved. One could stand with an apple seed in one's hand and imagine a future tree, with more apples and seeds, but go through a few generations and the maths get overwhelming. Others found the numbers exciting. In 1794, Erasmus Darwin thought reproduction was essentially caused by 'a wise superfluity', pointing out that young fish die in their countless millions, and they are more highly developed at the time of their demise than sperm. Then someone pointed out that fish were not wasted, and neither were plant seeds, because these became the food of other animals, while sperm were just lost. If sperm were so valuable, why did God waste so many millions of them? asked the insect anatomist, Lyonet, in 1742, and if sperm grow so rapidly in the uterus why don't they grow in the seminal fluid which is their 'native medium'? Turning to the philosophical, Lyonet asked, 'can we conceive that, in order to form our body, the least noble part of our being, God was willing to create so many hundreds of rational souls only to destroy them?' (quoted in Cole 1930:83). This raised another point which the best minds had questioned for centuries – when did the soul enter the body or potential body?

Ovism and spermism

Shortly before the discoveries in Delft, William Harvey, in 1651, stated that *omne vivum ex ovo* – all animals are produced from eggs, including man. This made him the first ovist, although he could not find a mammalian ovum. Harvey knew that an egg only becomes a live chick if it has been fertilized by a cockerel and deduced that the male in some way confers life. But he also knew of 'wind-eggs' – unfertilized eggs which produce live chickens – and stated that the female must therefore be credited with contributing 'form, species and soul'. However, because those wind-egg chickens were themselves infertile and unable to reproduce, Harvey was led to believe that the power of replication – the 'fructifying power' – was conferred by the father. Nevertheless, and although he couldn't prove it, Harvey was a rare advocate of a female role, saying women might have a 'more powerful right to be called the agent' of reproduction than men.

From a feminist perspective, ovism was not as revolutionary as it might first appear. Ovists could certainly argue that within the hypothetical 'ovum' there was a potential person waiting to get out, but everyone knew that intercourse and emission of semen had to happen first, so they had to assume that semen contributed something vital, if not the body itself. Ovism could imply that the ovum was a mini stillbirth unless touched by the mysterious 'vital impulse' of men, which could be interpreted as life force, soul or spirit. Spermists, on the other hand, could argue that sperm delivered the body, as well as life force, of the child.

The strongest scientific argument in favour of ovism was that early signs of visceral development could be observed in unfertilized eggs – Malpighi, Haller and Spallanzani saw it in chickens and frogs. Spallanzani, impressed at how a caterpillar egg can become a butterfly, thought frog's eggs contained everything necessary to form new frog bodies. Some were impressed by the fact that a female aphis can reproduce without a male, while others were misled into ovism by observations of dermoid cysts or ovarian pregnancies.

Spermism presented difficult questions. In 1717, Goelicke asked why these little tailed beings didn't produce a tailed animal when grown, and noted the theory didn't explain female sterility. In 1722, Maitre-Jan asked how bird's sperm could exist in the seminal fluid without drowning. He thought sperm must have fish-like characteristics, rather than bird ones, and thus actually transform rather than be preformed. To some, it seemed unlikely that sperm could be 'seed' because it was so similar in size and appearance when from very different species of animals. Others wanted to know what made sperm so different from the protozoa Leeuwenhoek found lurking in muddy puddles.

Many found spermism, which accepted that God should waste so many million precious seed, so incredible as to be impious. Ray, in 1693, thought it was much more likely that God would provide the seed in limited number – in the form of female eggs which 'may if need be, be all brought forth, and come to perfection'.

It might be thought that after the discovery of the Graafian follicle and sperm, someone would put one and one together and come to the conclusion that there was a shared parental contribution. At this time, however, people were too used to thinking in terms of a singular generant, while the epigenetic idea of a new creation was too mysterious to fathom.

Trying to find the elusive mammalian ovum, the foremost anatomist and physiologist of the eighteenth century, Haller, investigated forty sheep without success. It was commonly thought in Haller's time, and indeed almost a hundred years later, that intercourse caused the release, or formation, of the 'ovum'. Working in 1752, Haller thought that, on mating, a fluid was secreted and directed into the uterus, where it became mucoid and, later, produced the ovum by some process of coagulation.

Utter confusion characterized seventeenth- and eighteenth-century reproduction theory. In 1685 the teacher Drelincourt found it possible to collect 262 incorrect theories, and things had not improved a hundred years later, when Senebier wrote:

> In vain a host of ingenious and profound men have assembled observations on this important matter; in vain the boldest genius has analysed this capital question. The passing of centuries results only in a succession of errors, and whilst darkness the most profound has always obscured from the faculties of physiologists the secrets of generation, ideas the most incredible, contradictions the most flagrant, and travesties of nature the most incoherent have constituted the knowledge of those who flattered themselves on explaining the phenomena.
> (Serebeir, quoted in Cole 1930:118)

A resemblance to mother

Male-generant theories of reproduction needed to explain how children came to resemble their mothers and, given that the foetus spends nine months within the body of its mother, the possibilities for a maternal influence on the form of the child seemed many. Breast milk was another factor, and in the Italian universities of the fifteenth century, it was said to transmit physical characteristics of the woman, as well as intellectual and moral qualities.

Dutch professor of medicine, Hermann Boerhaave (1668–1738) wrote: 'The father communicates the embryo and first rudiments of life, the structure of the body being already determined and assigned in the animalcules of the male semen in all creatures, which yet receives some alteration according to the different species of animal or female from whence it is nourished (quoted in Cole 1930:85). This is not much more specific than the old farming idea that plants reflect the characteristics of the soil.

In 1714 Andry used 'uterine juices', possibly meaning amniotic fluid, to explain the intermediate character of hybrids: as told by F.J. Cole:

> Andry says that when the horse is paired with the ass, the progeny, on the emboitement theory, should resemble the father, since the form is determined by the male sex. The actual result, as is well known, is an intermediate, which has points in common with both parents. His explanation of this is that the juices which the spermatic worm of the horse encounters in the uterus of the ass, being adapted to produce a greater development of the ears than the juices which the same spermatic worm would have found in the uterus of one of its own species, it follows that the ears of the foetus will respond by a more vigorous growth. But the ears of the horse are not capable of all the growth to which such a nourishment is adapted, and therefore we should expect them to be longer than those of the horse, but shorter than those of the ass (Quoted in Cole 1930:73).

Jean Astruc, in 1762, said the sperm 'introduces itself into the pore or passage of the ovum, it is therein shaped, and, as it were, moulded; whence it is more or less stamped to the likeness of its mother, whose lineaments are impressed by the author of Nature on the hole or passage through which the animal enters the ovum' (quoted in Cole 1930:84). The tighter the fit in the 'passage', the more the child resembled its mother.

A later theory was 'pangenesis' – the idea that as blood travels around the body it picks up information in the form of 'gemmules'. These messengers of inheritance end their exhaustive journey in the genital system where they make up the generative male seed, semen, and the non-generative material of women – the menses or whatever. Long eyelashes and even an ear for music could be picked up in this way.

A resemblance to the mother could be attributed to the general – like 'movements of diverse humours' – or to the particular – her 'gemmules', her 'juices', her 'mould' or whatever. Anyone not convinced by these could turn to the mind.

In fifth-century Greece, Empedocles had said that 'the influence of the maternal imagination upon the embryo was so great that its formation could be guided and interfered with' (Needham 1959:29). Over the centuries there was a great deal of talk about 'the force of the mother's imagination', which sometimes meant a child resembled its mother because she particularly wanted to conceive at the time of intercourse; or because she was particularly desirous of the father at that time. Others believed a child looked like its mother if she had been suddenly frightened during early pregnancy.

Because even infertile men produce ejaculatory fluid, women generally got the blame for being 'barren'. If a woman produced only daughters it could be blamed on her mind, or on her faulty 'nourishment' – as if her 'soil' was too 'acid' or 'alkaline'. In 1685, Peyer blamed the occurrence of monster-children on the force of the mother's imagination or 'the machinations of the Devil, the foetus being deformed in the uterus as a punishment for sin' (Cole 1930:60).

The equalists

Equalists were few and far between and, although dual-parentage theories did emerge, they usually did so anonymously or posthumously, and in any case did not gain much favour. The mathematician René Descartes was one of these pragmatists, only allowing his *De la formation de l'animal* to be published after his death – in 1664, 24 years after he wrote it. He believed that male and female semen mixed, causing a 'fermentation of particles', the movement of which formed first the heart, and then the other embryonic parts. This was a very radical theory at the time and

Descartes feared the Catholic Church would come down heavily on him, as it had recently done on Galileo. In any case, his theory – a form of 'mechanistic epigenesis' – was unconvincing because it couldn't explain exactly how the foetus was formed.

In 1745, Maupertuis anonymously published a paper entitled 'Venus Physique', which pointed out that astronomers and chemists had recently proved the law of attraction and asked, 'Why should a cohesive force, if it exists in nature, Not have a role in the formation of animal bodies?' (Maupertuis [1745]1966:55–6; see also Roe 1981:13–15). He put forward the idea that both men and women produce seminal fluid which, when mixed, results in a developing embryo. This theory was met with much criticism partly because, as one critic, Remur, accused, the 'attraction' theory smacked of occultism. In 1759, more confident in the new discoveries of magnetic and chemical attraction, Wolff boldly suggested a new theory of epigenesis, which gained philosophical acceptance as the century drew to a close.

The question remained, however: was there a mammalian ovum? In 1797, William Cruikshank claimed to have found ova in the fallopian tubes of a rabbit but he was not believed, perhaps because, as it says in a biographical reference, 'he gave way to intemperance'. They thought he was drunk.

THE NINETEENTH CENTURY

At the turn of the nineteenth century, although no new embryological discoveries had been made, the scientific community had philosophically come around to the idea of epigenesis. It was from this perspective that J.M. Goode, writing in a *New Cyclopaedia* of 1813, reflected on the enduring and even recent success of spermism: 'The system of generation *ab animalculo maris* was still triumphantly maintained, and the feeble exertions of the few who had sense enough to oppose it was drowned in the multitudinous vociferation of their opponents' (Goode 1813: 'Generation', col. 5).

In 1824, Provost and Dumas proved that frog eggs are fertilized by the entry of spermatozoa, and epigenesis finally stood on solid ground. Preformation received a further blow in 1826, when Goeffrey proved that chick monsters could be produced if fertilized chicken eggs were incubated normally for three days and then shaken, perforated or coated with wax so no air could permeate the shell. The implication was that if development can be changed by such methods, it was not preformed.

Karl Ernst von Baer

The turning point for embryology came in spring 1827, when Karl Ernst von Baer looked down his microscope in Konigsberg, Germany, and discovered the mammalian ovum. The moment is recorded in his autobiography:

> Taking a single look through the instrument, I recoiled as if struck by lightning, because I saw a small, well-defined yellow yolk mass. I had to try and relax a while before I could work up enough courage to look again, as I was afraid I had been deluded by a phantom. Is it not strange that a sight which is expected, and indeed hoped for, should be frightening when it eventually materialises? (von Baer (1886) 1986:218)

Von Baer was modest about his discovery, attributing it to the 'conviction arrived at during my work with the chick', his eyesight – which 'made small pictures quite clear' – and good luck. He had chosen as the subject of his enquiry a dog – in which, apparently, the ovum is more clearly visible than in some other mammals.

The discovery disturbed the *status quo* and von Baer was met with '*altum silentum*' – silence. His paper, *De Ovi Mammalium et Hominis Genesi Epistola*, sold badly and the publisher declined to take on his next. In September 1828 von Baer attended a conference in Berlin and was surprised when:

> not a single one of the anatomists with whom I became acquainted even so much as mentioned my paper. The paper had been made available to the public as early as the middle of January, and it was highly unlikely that no one had heard of it, especially as I had taken care to have it sent to some of them.... I was too proud or too vain to bring up the subject myself in Berlin. Was my work regarded as a joke or a gross mistake? Or was the subject matter itself of too minor an importance to bother about? I really and truly did not know.... That the older men would not read my paper or, at least would not let it shake their convictions, I could well

> imagine. But that the younger participants, also remained silent – that I found disturbing. (von Baer (1886) 1986:225)

What happened at this conference was a microcosm of what was to happen in the macroscopic world of science later. To begin with, the participants were mesmerized into silence. They knew perfectly well the historical significance of von Baer's discovery and, indeed, that their own theories would have to change. Then, on the last day, one bold delegate came forward and asked the question everyone had on their minds: 'Could you not show us the mammalian ovum in the ovary?' (von Baer 1986:225) Von Baer willingly agreed and the janitor of the anatomical institute hurried off to prepare his bitch for the 'sacrifice'. 'A rather large number of anatomists' excitedly decamped to the dissection room, where von Baer duly provided the evidence. By the end of the afternoon, wrote von Baer, 'as far as I could make out, everyone seemed convinced, although I am certain that they had been rather doubtful earlier' (ibid.: 226). And so it was in the macroscopic world of science – a shocked, apparent indifference was followed by slow recognition, but eventual fame.

Von Baer's discovery made the idea of joint parentage a distinct possibility, but it was still too early in terms of both science and 'ethical considerations' for him to make that hypothesis:

> Perhaps we shall yet succeed in proving that the formative relations of the germinal vesicula and the spermatic animalcules correspond. We believe to have found a faint trace of the path to this secret. At present, however, it is still so dark and so little pursued that we do not risk proposing it. (quoted in Meyer 1956:116–17)

Nevertheless, von Baer felt himself out on a limb and, according to Meyer, after his discovery von Baer 'became distressed, distraught, spiritless and emaciated, and suffered constantly from nostalgia' (ibid.). Von Baer attributed his nervous breakdown to overwork and 'ethical considerations'.

Eleven years after von Baer's discovery Hausmann was still expanding on the old theory that the ovum coagulated from fluid, and there were those keen to agree with him, but this and other diversions would not deflect more than temporarily the path of truth which was, from now on, basically straight ahead.

Von Baer summarized his contribution within the context of the larger reproduction debate:

> The egg is ... an organised part of the maternal body, which almost always requires the intervention of the male procreative substance in order to develop under propitious conditions, into the corresponding animal according to its type. However, in which way and by what agency the male substance, having reached the egg that earlier was only a part and as such destined to die unless fertilised, now renders this egg capable of developing, that is, capable of becoming independent, is as yet not understood. (von Baer (1886) 1986:222)

The long road to understanding

Von Baer's 1827 discovery did not change things overnight. Twenty years later, Pouchet was fully prepared to accept that the ovum contained all the foetal material, but noted equally that it couldn't develop until man had delivered his mysterious 'vital impulse'. Establishing equal parentage would require dozens of crucial discoveries in the fields of embryology, cytology and genetics. It would take 50 years, after von Baer, to establish that reproduction involves the fusion of two single cells, and 129 years to establish that a person starts life with 46 chromosomes – 23 of which come from the father and 23 from the mother.

By 1839, division had been observed in the fertilized eggs of frogs, newts, fish, birds, hydroids, starfish, madusoids and rabbits, and by 1854, sperm had been seen to enter the corresponding egg in various species but not, as yet, in mammals. In 1861, Gegenbaur proved that the ovum is unicellular in all vertebrates, and in 1875 Beneden provided the first detailed description of the division of the fertilized mammalian ovum. In 1876, Oskar Hertwig became the first to recognize that the essential factor in fertilization is the fusion of sperm and ovum nuclei, and in 1879 Hermann Fol observed that a single sperm caused fertilization.

Running parallel to and interacting with embryological research were equally crucial developments in cytology and what we would later call genetics. In 1838 the German botanist Schleiden wrote that 'the lower plants all consist of one cell, while the higher ones are composed of [many]', and shortly afterwards

Schwann extended the theory to animals. In 1885 Kölliker described sperm as cellular in origin and nature and postulated that hereditary characteristics were transmitted by the cell nucleus. When the general statement of fact commonly called 'cell theory' came along, the knee-jerk reaction of some scientists was to declare that the ovum wasn't a cell because it didn't have a nucleus. It wasn't until 1861 that the ovum as proved to be unicellular – in vertebrates, at least. The sperm was confirmed to be a cell in 1885. In 1892 Weismann anticipated the chromosomal basis of inheritance with his 'germ plasm' theory, and soon after the turn of the twentieth century, Boveri proved it.

In 1891 Henking was the first to see the accessory chromosomes and in 1902 McClung demonstrated that they were the determinants of gender. In 1900 three botanists independently recognized the importance of Mendel's work on the hereditary traits of garden peas, which had been written 35 years previously but dismissed as irrelevant by Von Nageli – a distinguished botanist at the time. With the turn of the twentieth century, the front line in research moved from cellular biology into molecular biology. In 1909 Johannsen coined the term 'gene', which was adopted by Morgan and others to describe the sub-units of chromosomes. Working particularly with the fruit fly *drosophila*, in 1915 Morgan showed that genes are responsible for identifiable, hereditary traits.

Correct theory had begun in 1827 with von Baer's discovery of the mammalian ovum, and by 1900 science had enough evidence to say that there is equal parental contribution to reproduction. Important details kept coming in, such as the demonstration that the normal number of chromosomes in humans is 46, by Tjio and Levan in 1956. But if someone required actual photographic proof that human beings reproduce in much the same way as frogs or sea urchins, they had to wait until IVF experimentation on humans and, in 1960, a slim volume of photomicrographs entitled *Ovum Humanum*, by Dr Landrum Shettles. For the first time, there it was for all to see – human sperm entering the human ovum, and the subsequent cell division that would lead to a foetus.

HOW BIOLOGY BECAME DESTINY

When, in the long road to understanding, a particular person chose to see the emerging truth of female generativity very much depended on their degree of prejudice against it. There were many commentators who took any available chance to continue the notion that women are basically inferior. In 1883, for example, W.K. Brooks in *The Law of Heredity* wrote, 'One of the most remarkable and suggestive of the laws of variation' was that the exclusively male parts were 'very much more variable' (Brooks 1883:257) than the female parts. It wasn't clear whether he was saying that penises differ from one another in size and shape more than vaginas do, or that each individual penis can vary its size and shape considerably. But, according to Brooks, 'the male element is the originating and the female the perpetuating factor; the ovum is the conservative, the male cell progressive'. This apparently affected the brain:

> if the male organism is the conservative organism, to which is intrusted the keeping of all that has been gained during the past history of the race, it must follow that the female mind is a storehouse filled with the instincts, habits, intuitions, and laws of conduct which have been gained by past experience. The male organism, on the contrary, being the variable organism, the originating element in the process of evolution, the male mind must have the power of extending experience over new fields, and, by comparison and generalisation, of discovering new laws of nature.... (Brooks 1883:257)

For thousands of years, using 'comparison and generalisation', science conspired to belittle the contribution of women. From misconceptions about her blood, veins, ovaries, ovum, menses and vagina, woman's inferiority had been 'proved' and further defined.

When reproductive biology couldn't do the job, something else was found - her lack of facial hair, the shape of her abdomen, her 'missing five ounces' of brain weight, and even the fact that she seldom goes bald. There was never a shortage of theories. Men seemed desperate to find anything which could prove their superiority, perhaps because they had an inferiority complex as far as the generation of life was concerned. In 1794 Erasmus Darwin, Charles's learned grandfather, reasoned that because men are bigger they 'should contribute as much or more towards the reproduction of the species' (Darwin 1794). As women already did so much in terms of nourishment and warmth, men must contribute something more valuable – life itself. Perhaps it only seemed fair.

A COMPLICATED ISSUE: THE INVISIBLE REVOLUTION

Late nineteenth-century embryology involved more than the facts of reproduction. The white men of science were concerned to know where they stood, not only in relation to white women, but in relation to animals, God and black people. Charles Darwin caused a furore in 1859 when, in *The Origin of Species*, he suggested that men and women were descended from apes, and embryology disturbed things further by showing that human embryos look at first like fish, then like reptiles, before taking on their human form – thereby strangely following an evolutionary course. Human embryos also look remarkably similar, at an early stage, to the embryos of many other animals.

Science moved inexorably forward, away from the fundamentals – such as where did the seed come from – and into the minuscule details. As the jigsaw fell into place, the textbooks were rewritten presenting the new facts and omitting the long story that led to them. We came to have the impression that, although our ancestors didn't know the precise details of gene transference, they believed as we now did, that human reproduction was accomplished by the fusion of both male and female generative 'seed', which we now called ovum and sperm. In fact, they knew nothing of the sort.

Several factors converged to make invisible the profound change that happened in reproductive thinking, particularly in terms of women's new-found role. The 'facts of life' were revealed by many embryological discoveries during the course of a century or more so it was difficult to identify a specific date at which the revolution took place. Women were absent from the scientific scene which is why, perhaps, nobody came forward to put the embryological discoveries of the nineteenth century in a feminist context; and if a man made it the subject of his after-dinner speech at the Royal Society, it was likely to alienate him from his sexist peers.

Embryology involves sex and creation which makes it open to theological, philosophical and sexual sensitivities. Of all the branches of science, it was most liable to be left out of discussions – at public talks, in drawing rooms or in front of children. Somehow, the relevant books didn't get into general circulation. Information had to come from science but during the Victorian era at least, as Cole (1930) says, 'a gulf was fixed between the secluded specialists who discussed these matters in profound or at least technical language and a public who were educated on moral principles laid down 2,000 or more years ago'.

Life, tradition, went on as usual. The twentieth century brought better education, especially for women, but without a knowledge of embryological history, it was easy to get the mistaken impression that the basic facts of life – that there are two generative seeds and fusion – had always been understood in European culture.

NOTES

1 Dr Landrum Shettles, *Ovum Humanum*, 1960.
2 I am grateful to C.D. Darlington for this observation: (Darlington 1964:66).
3 As *erythrinus* means 'red', it is thought Aristotle referred to *Serranus anthius*, a fish that is a brilliant red.
4 Malachi 4:6, regarding Elijah: 'And he shall turn the heart of the fathers to the children, and the heart of the children to their fathers, lest I come and smite the earth with a curse.'
5 Raghib, *Safinat*, ed. Bulaq (Cairo, 1286h.), p. 15 ff.

BIBLIOGRAPHY

CHAPTER I

Banal, I. and Verdery, K. 1995. *National Character and National Ideology in Interwar Eastern Europe*, New Haven, Yale Centre for International Studies.

Barnard, A. 1994. 'Rules and prohibitions: the form and content of human kinship', in T. Ingold, ed., *Companion Encyclopedia of Anthropology: Humanity, Culture and Social Life*. London, Routledge.

Barth, F. 1987. *Cosmologies in the Making: A Generative Approach to Cultural Variation in inner New Guinea*, Cambridge, Cambridge University Press.

Bloch, M. and Parry, J., eds. 1982. *Death and the Regeneration of Life*, Cambridge, Cambridge University Press.

Bourdieu, P. 1977. *Outline of a Theory of Practice*, trans. Richard Nice, Cambridge, Cambridge University Press.

Carsten, J. 1992. 'The process of childbirth and becoming related among Malays in Pulau Langkawi', in G. Aijmer, ed., *Coming into Existence*, Institute of Advanced Studies, University of Gothenburg.

Daniel, V. 1984. *Fluid Signs: Being a Person the Tamil Way*, Berkeley, University of California Press.

Delaney, C. 1986. 'The meaning of paternity and the virgin birth debate', *Man* 21 (3), 494–513.

—— 1991. *The Seed and the Soil: Gender and Cosmology in a Turkish Village,* Berkeley, University of California Press.

Dube, L 1986. 'Seed and earth: the symbolism of biological reproduction and sexual relations of production', in L. Dube, E. Leacock and S. Ardener, eds, *Visibility and Power: Essays on Women in Society and Development*, Delhi, Oxford University Press.

Du Boulay, J. 1991. 'Cosmos and gender in village Greece', in P. Loizos and E. Papataxiarchis, eds, *Gender and Kinship in Modern Greece*, Princeton, Princeton University Press.

Engels, F. 1941 *The Origin of the Family, Private Property and the State*. London: Lawrence and Wishart. (German Original, 1884).

Frazer, J.G. 1890 *The Golden Bough: A Study in Magic and Religion*, London, McMillan.

Goody, E. 1982. *Parenthood and Social Reproduction: Fostering and Occupational Roles in West Africa*, Cambridge, Cambridge University Press.

Hocart, A.M. 1927. *Kingship*, London, Oxford University Press.

Ingold, T. 1994. 'Introduction to social life', in T. Ingold, ed., *Companion Encyclopedia of Anthropology: Humanity, Culture and Social Life*, London, Routledge.

Leach, E. 1966. 'Virgin birth', *Proceedings of the Royal Anthropological Institute for 1966*, 39–49.

Leach, E. 1969. *Genesis as Myth and Other Essays*, London, Cape.

Lévi-Strauss, C. 1963. *Totemism*, trans R. Needham, Boston, Beacon.

—— 1966. *The Savage Mind*, Chicago, Chicago University Press.

—— 1969. *The Elementary Structures*, Boston, Beacon Press.

LiPuma, E. 1988. *The Gift of Kinship*, Cambridge, Cambridge University Press.

MacCormack, C. and Strathern, M. eds. 1980. *Nature, Culture and Gender*, Cambridge, Cambridge University Press.

McKnight, D. 1975. 'Men, women, and other animals: taboo and purification among the Wik-mungan', in R. Willis, ed., *The Interpretation of Symbolism*, London, Malaby Press, 77–97.

Malinowski, B. 1932. *The Sexual Life of Savages in North Western Melanesia*, London, Routledge and Kegan Paul.

Marx, K. and Engels, F. 1848. *The Communist Manifesto*. Reprinted in K. Marx and F. Engels, 1968, *Selected Works*, New York, International Publishers.

Morgan, L.H. 1869. *Systems of Affinity and Consanguinity in the Family*, Washington, D.C., Smithsonian Institute.

Needham, R. 1971, *Rethinking Kinship and Marriage*, Association of Social Anthropologists Monographs in Social Anthropology, London, Tavistock Publications.

Ortner, S.B. 1972. 'Is female to male as nature is to culture?' reprinted in M.Z. Rosaldo and L. Lamphere, eds, *Women, Culture and Society*, Stanford, Stanford University Press.

Ortner, S.B. and Whitehead, H., eds. 1981. *Sexual Meanings: The Cultural Construction of Gender and Sexuality*, Cambridge, Cambridge University Press.

Peters, E. 1967. 'Some structural aspects of the feud among the camel-herding Bedouin of Cyrenaica', *Africa* 37, 261–82.

Pina-Cabral, J. 1986. *Sons of Adam, Daughters of Eve: The Peasant Worldview of the Alto Minho*, Oxford, Clarendon.

Poole, Fitz John Porter. 1981. 'Transforming "natural" women: female ritual leaders and gender ideology among Bimin-Kuskusmin', in S.B. Ortner and H. Whitehead, eds, *Sexual Meanings: The Cultural Construction of Gender and Sexuality*, Cambridge, Cambridge University Press.

Sahlins, M. 1976. *The Use and Abuse of Biology: An Anthropological Critique of Sociobiology*, Ann Arbor, University of Michigan Press.

Sanders, T. 1997. 'Rainmaking, gender and power in Ihanzu, Tanzania, 1885-1995' unpublished doctoral thesis, London School of Economics.

Schneider, D. 1984. *A Critique of the Study of Kinship*, Ann Arbor, University of Michigan Press.

Spiro, M.E. 1968. 'Virgin birth, parthenogenesis, and physiological paternity: an essay on cultural interpretation', *Man* 3 2, 242–61.

Strathern, M. 1988. *The Gender of the Gift. Problems with Women and Problems with Society in Melanesia*, Berkeley, University of California Press.

Tonkinson, R. 1978. 'Semen versus spirit-child in Western Desert culture', in L. Hiatt, ed., *Australian Aboriginal Concepts*, Canberra, Australian Institute of Aboriginal Studies.

CHAPTER 2

Ahern, Emily Martin. 1979. 'The problem of efficacy: strong and weak illocutionary acts', *Man* (N.S.) 14, 1–17.

Astuti, Rita. 1993. 'Food for pregnancy: procreation, marriage and images of gender among the Vezo of western Madagascar', *Social Anthropology* 1, 277–90.

—— 1995a. *People of the Sea: Descent and Identity among the Vezo of Western Madagascar*, Cambridge, Cambridge University Press.

—— 1995b. "The Vezo are not a kind of people": identity, difference and "ethnicity" among a fishing people of western Madagascar', *American Ethnologist* 22, 464–82.

Austin, J.L. 1962. *How To Do Things with Words*, London, Oxford University Press.

Baré, Jean François. 1977. *Pouvoirs des Vivants, Langage des Morts: Idéo-Logiques Sakalave,* Paris, Maspero.

Barnett, Steve. 1976. 'Coconuts and gold: relational identity in a South Indian subcaste', *Contributions to Indian Sociology* (N.S.) 10, 133–56.

Bloch, Maurice. 1971. *Placing the Dead: Tombs, Ancestral Villages and Kinship Organization in Madagascar*, London, Seminar Press.

—— 1981. 'Hierarchy and equality in Merina kinship', *Ethnos* 46, 5–18.

—— 1987. 'Descent and sources of contradiction in representations of women and kinship', in J.F. Collier and S.J. Yanagisako, eds, *Gender and Kinship*, Stanford, Calif., Stanford University Press, 324–37.

—— 1993. 'Zafimaniry birth and kinship theory', *Social Anthropology* 1 (1b), 119–32.

Bourdieu, Pierre. 1977. *Outline of a Theory of Practice*, Cambridge, University Press.

Busby, Cecilia. 1997a. 'Of marriage and marriageability: gender and Dravidian kinship', *Journal of the Royal Anthropological Institute* (N.S.) 3, 21–42.

—— 1997b. 'Permeable and partible persons: a comparative analysis of gender and body in south India and Melanesia', *Journal of the Royal Anthropological Institute* (N.S.) 3, 261–78.

Carsten, Janet. 1995. 'The substance of kinship and the heat of the hearth: feeding, personhood and relatedness among Malays of Pulau Langkawi'. *American Ethnologist* 22, 223–41.

Clay, Brenda J. 1977. *Pinikindu: Maternal Nurture, Paternal Substance*, Chicago, University of Chicago Press.

Daniel, E. Valentine. 1984. *Fluid Signs: Being a Person the Tamil Way*, Berkeley, University of California Press.

Feeley-Harnik, Gillian. 1991. *A Green Estate: Restoring Indepen-*

dence in Madagascar, Washington, D.C., Smithsonian Institution Press.
—— n.d. 'Ancestry, birth, and the custody of children: comparative perspectives from Madagascar', *American Ethnologist*, forthcoming.
Franklin, Sarah. 1997. *Embodied Progress: A Cultural Account of Assisted Conception,* London, Routledge.
Gibson, Thomas. 1985. 'The sharing of substance versus the sharing of activity among the Buid', *Man* (N.S.) 20, 391–411.
Howell, Signe and Melhuus, Marit. 1993. 'The study of kinship; the study of person: a study of gender?', in T. del Valle, ed., *Gendered Anthropology*, London, Routledge, 38–53.
Huntington, Richard. 1988. *Gender and Social Structure in Madagascar*. Bloomington, Indiana University Press.
Inden, Ronald B. and Nicholas, Ralph W. 1977. *Kinship in Bengali Culture*, Chicago, University of Chicago Press.
Kottak, Conrad P. 1980. *The Past in the Present: History, Ecology and Cultural Variation in Highland Madagascar*, Ann Arbor, University of Michigan Press.
Lambek, Michael. 1992. 'Taboo as a cultural system among Malagasy speakers', *Man* (N.S.) 27, 245–66.
Latour, Bruno. 1993. *We Have Never Been Modern*, Cambridge, Mass., Harvard University Press.
LiPuma, Edward. 1988. *The Gift of Kinship: Structure and Practice in Maring Social Organization*, Cambridge, University Press.
McGilvray, Dennis. 1982. 'Mukkuvar Vannimai: Tamil caste and matriclan ideology, in Batticaloa, Sri Lanka', in D. McGilvray, ed., *Caste Ideology and Interaction,* Cambridge, Cambridge, University Press.
Morris, Rosalind C. 1995. 'All made up: performance theory and the new anthropology of sex and gender', *Annual Review of Anthropology*, 24, 567–92.
Needham, Rodney. 1971. 'Remarks on the analysis of kinship and marriage', in R. Needham, ed., *Rethinking Kinship and Marriage*, London, Tavistock, 1–34.
Peletz, Michael G. 1995. 'Kinship studies in the late twentieth century', *Annual Review of Anthropology* 24, 343–72.
Sahlins, Marshall. 1985. *Islands of History*, Chicago, University of Chicago Press.

Scheffler, Harold W. 1991. 'Naturalism and sexism in the study of kinship', in M. di Leonardo, ed., *Gender at the Crossroads of Knowledge*, Berkeley, University of California Press.

Schneider, David M. 1968. *American Kinship: A Cultural Account*, Englewood Cliffs, N.J., Prentice Hall.

—— 1972. 'What is kinship all about?', in P. Reining, ed., *Kinship Studies in the Morgan Centennial Year,* Washington, D.C., Anthropological Society of Washington, 32–63.

—— 1976. 'Notes toward a theory of culture', in K. Basso and H. Selby, eds, *Meaning in Anthropology*, Albuquerque, University of New Mexico Press, 197–220.

—— 1980. *American Kinship*. 2nd edn. Chicago, University of Chicago Press.

—— 1984. *A Critique of the Study of Kinship*. Ann Arbor, University of Michigan Press.

Schneider, Daniel M. and Richard Handler. 1995. *Schneider on Schneider: The Conversion of the Jews and other Anthropological Stories*, Durham, N.C., Duke University Press.

Strathern, Andrew. 1973. 'Kinship, descent and locality: some New Guinea examples', in J. Goody, ed., *The Character of Kinship*, Cambridge, University Press, 21–33.

Strathern, Marilyn. 1995. 'Displacing knowledge: technology and the consequences for kinship', in F.D. Ginsburg and R. Rapp, eds, *Conceiving the New World Order*, Berkeley, University of California Press, 346–63.

—— 1996. 'Cutting the network', *Journal of the Royal Anthropological Institute* (N.S.) 2, 517–35.

Tambiah, Stanley J. [1981] 1985. 'A performative approach to ritual', in *Culture, Thought and Social Action*, Cambridge, Mass., Harvard University Press, 123–66.

Thomas, Philip. 1995. 'Of houses, hearths and granaries: some aspects of gender among the Temanambondro of southeast Madagascar', *Indonesia Circle* 67 (special issue, 'Gender and the sexes in the Indonesian archipelago', eds. L. Summers and W.D. Wilder).

—— 1996. 'Place, Person and Ancestry among the Temanambondro of Southeast Madagascar', unpublished PhD thesis, University of London.

—— 1997. 'The water that blesses, the river that flows: place and the ritual imagination among the Temanambondro of southeast Madagascar', in J.J. Fox, ed., *The Poetic Power of Place: Com-*

parative Perspectives on Austronesian Ideas of Locality, Canberra, Department of Anthropology, Research School of Pacific Studies, the Australian National University.
Wagner, Roy. 1967. *The Curse of Souw: Principles of Daribi Clan Definition and Alliance,* Chicago, University of Chicago Press.
Weiner, James F. 1982. 'Substance, siblingship and exchange: aspects of social structure in New Guinea', *Social Analysis* 11, 3–34.
Weston, Kath. 1995. 'Forever is a long time: romancing the real in gay kinship ideologies', in S.J. Yanagisako and C. Delaney, eds, *Naturalizing Power*. New York, Routledge, 87–110.
Witherspoon, Gary. 1978. *Navajo Kinship and Marriage*, Chicago, University of Chicago Press.
Yanagisako, Sylvia J. 1978. 'Variance in American kinship: implications for cultural analysis', *American Ethnologist* 5, 15–29.
Yanagisako, Sylvia J. and Collier, Jane F. 1987. 'Toward a unified analysis of gender and kinship', in J.F. Collier and S.J. Yanagisako, eds, *Gender and Kinship*, Stanford, Calif., Stanford University Press, 14–50.

CHAPTER 3

Aijmer, G. ed. *Coming into Existence*, Gothenberg, Institute of Advanced Studies, University of Gothenberg.
Astuti, R. 1992. '"*Learning to be Vezo'. The Construction of the Person Among Fishing People of Western Madagascar*', PhD thesis, University of London.
Beidelman, T.O. 1964. 'Pig (Guluwe):. An Essay on Ngulu Sexual Symbolism and Ceremony', *Southwestern Journal of Anthropology* 20, 359–93.
—— 1967. *The Matrilineal Peoples of Eastern Tanzania*, London, International African Institute.
—— 1986. *Moral Imagination in Kaguru Modes of Thought*, Bloomington, Indiana University Press.
Bloch, M. 1975. 'Property and the end of affinity', in M. Bloch ed., *Marxist Analyses and Social Anthropology,* London, Malaby, 203–22.
—— 1992. 'Birth and the beginning of social life among the Zafimaniry of Madagascar', in G. Aijmer ed., *Coming into*

Existence, Gothenburg, Institute of Advanced Studies, University of Gothenburg.70–90.

Bourdieu, P. 1977. *Outline of a Theory of Practice*, Cambridge, Cambridge University Press.

Boyer, P. 1990. *Tradition as Truth and Communication. A Cognitive Description of Traditional Discourse*, Cambridge, Cambridge University Press.

Brain, J.L. 1978. 'Symbolic rebirth: The mwali rite among the Luguru of eastern Tanzania', *Africa* 48 (2), 177–88.

Bryceson, D.F. 1995. 'Gender relations in rural Tanzania: power politics or cultural consensus', in C. Creighton and C. Omari, eds, *Gender, Family and Household in Tanzania*, Aldershot, Avebury, 37–69.

Caplan, A.P. 1976. 'Boys' circumcision and girls' puberty rites among the Swahili of Mafia Island, Tanzania', *Africa* 46 (1), 21–33.

Carsten, J. 1992. 'The process of childbirth and becoming related among Malays in Pulau Langkawi', in G. Aijmer ed., *Coming into Existence*, Gothenburg, Institute of Advanced Studies, University of Gothenburg, 19–46.

Clark, M. 1984. 'Woman headed households and poverty: insights from Kenya'. *Signs* 10 (2), 338–54.

Evans-Pritchard, E.E. 1940. *The Nuer. A Description of the Modes of Livelihood and Political Institutions of a Nilotic People*, Oxford, Oxford University Press.

Falk Moore, S. 1986. *Social Facts and Fabrications: 'Customary' Law on Kilimanjaro, 1880–1980*, Cambridge, Cambridge University Press.

Fortes, M. 1953. 'The structure of unilineal descent groups,' *American Anthropologist*, 55 (1), 17–41.

Geertz, C. 1973. 'Religion as a cultural system', in *The Interpretation of Cultures*, London, Fontana, 87–125.

Gluckman, M. 1950. 'Kinship and marriage among the Lozi', in A.R. Radcliffe-Brown and D. Forde, eds, *African Systems of Kinship and Marriage*, London, Oxford University Press, 166–206.

Green, M. 1993. 'The construction of "religion" and the perpetuation of "tradition" among Pogoro Catholics, southern Tanzania', unpublished PhD thesis, University of London.

—— 1996. 'Medicines and the embodiment of substances among Pogoro Catholics, southern Tanzania', *Journal of the Royal Anthropological Institute*, (N.S.) 2, 1–14.

Guyer, J.L. and Peters, P.E. 1987. 'Conceptualising the household: issues of theory, method and application', *Development and Change* 18, 197–214.

Harris, O. 1981. 'Households as natural units', in K. Young *et al.*, eds, *Of Marriage and the Market,* London, CSE Books, 49–68.

Jilek-Aal, L. 1976. 'Kifafa: 'A Tribal Disease in an East African Bantu Population', in J. Westermayer, ed., *Anthropology and Mental Health*, The Hague, Mouton.

Kratz, C. 1994. *Affecting Performance. Meaning, Movement, and Experience in Okiek Women's Initiation*, Washington, D.C., Smithsonian Institution Press.

MacCormack, C. 1982. 'Health, fertility and birth in Moyamba District, Sierra Leone', in C. MacCormack, ed., *Ethnography of Fertility and Birth*, London, Academic Press, 115–39.

Maghimbi, S. 1990. 'Rural development policy and planning in Tanzania', PhD Thesis, London University.

Molyneaux, M. 1977. 'Androcentrism in Marxist anthropology', *Critique of Anthropology* 3 (9, 10), 55–81.

Moore, H.L. 1995. *A Passion for Difference: Essays in Anthropology and Gender*, Cambridge, Polity.

Omari, C.K. 1995. 'Decision-making and the household: Case studies from Tanzania', in C. Creighton and C.K. Omari, eds, *Gender, Family and Household in Tanzania,* Aldershot, Avebury, 203–21.

Parkin, D. 1980. 'Kind bridewealth and hard cash: eventing a structure', in J.L. Comaroff, ed., *The Meaning of Marriage Payments*, London, Academic Press, 197–221.

Parkin, D. and Nyamwaya, D. 1987. 'Introduction: transformations of African marriage: change and choice', in D. Parkin and D. Nyamwaya, eds, *Transformations of African Marriage,* London, International African Institute, 1–16.

Poewe, K.O. 1978. 'Matriliny in the throes of change: kinship, descent and marriage in Luapula, Zambia', *Africa* 48 (3), 205–19 and 48 (4), 353–67.

Radcliffe-Brown, A.R. 1950. 'Introduction', in A.R. Radcliffe-Brown and D. Forde, eds, *African Systems of Kinship and Marriage,* London, Oxford University Press, 1–85.

Ranger, T.O. 1983. 'The invention of tradition in colonial Africa', in E. Hobsbawm and T.O. Ranger, eds, *The Invention of Tradition*, Cambridge, Cambridge University Press, 211–62.

Richards, A.I.1939. *Land Labour and Diet in Northern Rhodesia. An Economic Study of the Bemba Tribe,* London, Oxford University Press.

—— 1950. 'Some types of family structure amongst the central Bantu', in A.R. Radcliffe-Brown and D. Forde eds, *African Systems of Kinship and Marriage,* London, Oxford University Press, 207–51.

—— 1982. *Chisungu. A Girl's Initiation Ceremony among the Bemba of Zambia,* London, Routledge.

Schneider, D.M. 1984. *A Critique of the Study of Kinship*, Ann Arbor, University of Michigan Press.

Sender, J. and Smith, S. 1990. *Poverty, Class and Gender in Rural Africa: A Tanzanian Case Study*, London, Routledge.

Strathern, A. 1973. 'Kinship, descent and locality. Some New Guinea examples', in J. Goody, ed., *The Character of Kinship*, Cambridge, Cambridge University Press.

Swantz, M.L. 1966. *Religious and magical rites of Bantu women in Tanzania*, dissertation, University of Dar es Salaam.

—— 1970. *Ritual and Symbol in Transitional Zaramo Society, with Special Reference to Women,* Uppsala, Scandinavian Institute of African Studies.

Turner, V.W. 1968. *The Drums of Affliction. A Study of Religious Processes among the Ndembu of Zambia*, Oxford, Clarendon Press.

Wilson, M. 1950. 'Nyakyusa kinship', in A.R. Radcliffe-Brown and D. Forde, eds, *African Systems of Kinship and Marriage,* London, Oxford University Press, 111–39.

—— 1957. *Rituals of Kinship among the Nyakyusa,* London, Oxford University Press.

Worsely, P. 1956). 'The kinship system of the Tallensi. A reevaluation', *Journal of the Royal Anthropological Institute*, 86, 37–75.

CHAPTER 4

Abercrombie, Thomas. 1998. *Pathways of Memory and Power: Ethnography and History among an Andean People*. Madison, University of Wisconsin Press.

Albó, Xavier, 1975 *La Paradoja Aymara: Solidaridad y Faccionalismo*, La Paz, CIPCA.

—— 1985. *Desafios de la Solidaridad Aymara*, La Paz, CIPCA.

Albó, X., Greaves, T. and Sandoval, G. 1987. *Chukiyawu: La Cara Aymara de La Paz*, iv, Nuevos Lazos con el Campo. La Paz, CIPCA.

Allen, Catherine. 1988. *The Hold Life Has: Coca and Cultural Identity in an Andean Community*. Washington, D.C., Smithsonian Institution Press.

Arnold, Denise. 1989. 'Matrilineal practice in a patrilineal setting: rituals and metaphors of kinship in an Andean ayllu'. unpublished Ph.D. thesis, University of London.

Arnold, Denise and de Dio Yapita, Juan. 1996. 'Los caminos de género en el ayllu Qaqachaka: los saberes femeninos y los discursos textuales alternativos', in Silvia Rivera, ed., *Ser mujer indígena, chola o birlocha en la Bolivia (postcolonial) de los 90*, La Paz, Subsecretaría de Género/CID pp.303-392

Bastien, Joseph. 1978. *Mountain of the Condor*, St Paul, West Publishing Co.

van den Berg, Hans. 1990. *La Tierra no da asi nomás: Los Ritos Agrícolas en la Religión de los Aymara-Cristianos*, La Paz, HISBOL.

van den Berghe, Pierre and Primov, George. 1977. *Inequality in the Peruvian Andes: Class and Ethnicity in Cuzco*, Columbia, Mo., University of Missouri Press.

Bloch, Maurice. 1992. 'Birth and the beginning of social life among the Zafiminiry of Madagascar', in Göran Aijmer, ed., *Coming into Existence: Birth and Metaphors of Birth,* Göteborg, IASSA, 71–91.

Bloch, Maurice and Guggenheim, S. 1981. 'Compadrazgo, baptism and the symbolism of a second birth', *Man*, 16, (3), 376–86.

Canessa, Andrew. 1993. 'The Politics of Pacha', unpublished PhD dissertation, University of London.

—— 1997. 'Chachawarmi: negociando (des)igualdades de genero en una aldea Aymara Boliviana', in Denise Arnold, ed., *Nuevas Direcciones en los Estudios Andinos*, La Paz, ILCA/CID.

Carter, W. and Mamani, M. 1982. *Irpa Chico: Individuo y Comunidad en la Cultura Aymara,* La Paz, Bolivia, Juventud.

Delaney, Carol, 1991. *The Seed and the Soil: Gender and Cosmology in Turkish Village Society*, Berkeley, University of California Press.

Friedlander, J. 1975. *Being Indian in Hueyapan: A Study of Forced Identity in Contemporary Mexico*, New York, St Martin's Press.

Gose, Peter. 1994. *Deathly Waters and Hungry Mountains*, Toronto, Toronto University Press.

Harris, Olivia 1980. 'The power of signs: gender, culture and the wild in the Bolivian Andes', in C. MacCormack and M. Strathern, eds, *Nature, Culture and Gender*, Cambridge, Cambridge University Press, 70–94.

—— 1982. 'The dead and the devils among the Bolivian Laymi', in M. Bloch and J. Parry, eds, *Death and the Regeneration of Life*, Cambridge, Cambridge University Press, 45–73.

—— 1995. 'Ethnic identity and market relations: indians and mestizos in the Andes', in O. Harris, B. Larson and E. Tandeter, eds, *Ethnicity and Markets in the Andes: Indian Economies and Commercial Adaptations 16th–20th Centuries*, Durham N.C. and London, Duke University Press.

Isbell, Billy Jean. 1978. *To Defend Ourselves: Ecology and Ritual in an Andean Village*, Austin, University of Texas Press.

Kurtz, Stanley. 1992. *All the Mothers are One: Hindu India and the Cultural Reshaping of Psychoanlysis,* New York, Columbia University Press.

Mayer, Enrique. 1975. 'Reciprocity, self-sufficiency and market relations in a contemporary community in the central Andes of Peru', *Latin American Studies Dissertation* Series no. 72, Ithaca, Cornell University Press.

Orlove, Benjamin. 1998. 'Down to earth: race and substance in the Andes', *Bulletin of Latin American Research* 17, (2), 207–222.

Saignes, Thierry. 1993. 'Borracheras Andinas, porqué los indios ebrios hablan en español?', in T. Saignes, *La Experiencia de lo Sagrado en los Andes*, La Paz, HISBOL/IFEA.

Sallnow, Michael. 1987. *Pilgrims of the Andes*, Washington D.C., Smithsonian Institute Press.

Skar, Harald. 1982. *The Warm Valley People*, Oslo, Universitetsforlaget.

Spedding, Allison. 1989. 'Wachu Wachu: coca cultivation and Aymara identity in the yunkas of La Paz (Bolivia)', unpublished PhD thesis, University of London.

Wade, Peter. 1997. *Race and Ethnicity in Latin America*, London, Pluto.

Weismantel, Mary. 1997. 'White cannibals: fantasies of racial violence in the Andes', *Identities* 4 (1), 9–43.

CHAPTER 5

Adatrechtbundel III. 1910. *Rapport over de adat kebiasaan, uitgebracht door een inlandsche comissie (1896).* Serie M: 'Minahasa' no 1:1–113, Commissie voor het Adat-recht, Koninklijk Instituut voor de Taal[, Land-en Volkenkunde van Nederlandsch-Indië, The Hague, Martinus Nijhoff. (Special Malay version compiled by three Minahasan chiefs).

Anderson, B. 1972. 'The idea of power in Japanese culture', in C. Holt, ed., *Culture and Politics in Indonesia*, Ithaca, Cornell University Press.

Atkinson, J.M. 1996. 'Quizzing the Sphinx. Reflections on mortality in Central Sulawesi', in L.J. Sears, ed., *Fantasizing the Feminine in Indonesia*, London, Duke University Press.

Babcock, T. G. 1986. *The Religion and Cultural Identity in Kampung Java Tandano*, Yogyakarta, University of Gadjah Mada.

Bakhuitzen van den Brink, C. [1880] 1915. 'De Inlandsche Burgers in de Molukken', *Bijdragen tot de Taal-, Land- en Volkenkunde van Nederlandsch-Indië* 70, 595-649, Batavia, Martinus Nijhoff.

Bemmelen, S. van. 1992. 'The marriage of Minahasa women in the period of 1861–1933', in E. Locher-Scholten and A. Niehof, eds, *Indonesian Women in Focus*, Leiden, KITLV Press.

Bloch, M. 1992. 'Birth and the beginning of 'Social Life' among the Zafimaniry of Madagascar', in G. Aijmer, ed., *Coming into Existence: Birth and Metaphors of Birth*, Göteberg, Institute of Advanced Studies in Social Anthropology, University of Gothenberg.

Boomgaard, P. 1993. 'The development of colonial health care in Java; an exploratory introduction, *Bijdragen tot de Taal – Land – en Volkenkunde*, 149, 77–93.

—— 1996. 'Dutch medicine in Asia, 1600–1900', in D. Arnold ed., *Warm Climates and Western Medicine: The Emergence of Tropical Medicine, 1500–1900*, Clio Medica, Atlanta/Amsterdam, Rodopi.

Bowen, J.R. 1993. *Muslims through Discourse. Religion and Ritual in Gayo Society*, Princeton, N.J., Princeton University Press.

Bucholt, H. 1994. 'The impact of the Christian mission on processes of social differentiation', in H. Buchholt and U. Mai, eds, *Continuity, Change and Aspirations: Social and Cultural Life in Minahasa, Indonesia*, Singapore, ISEAS.

Carpentier Alting, J.H. 1902. 'Het gewoonte-recht in de Minahasa', *De Indische gids* 23, 129–44.

Carsten, J. 1991. 'Children in between: fostering and the process of kinship on Pulau Langkawi, Malaysia', *Man (N.S.)* 26, 425–44.

—— 1992. 'The process of childbirth and becoming related among Malays in Pulau Langkawi', in G. Aijmer, ed., *Coming into Existence: Birth and Metaphors in Birth*, Gothenburg. Institute of Advanced Studies in Social Anthropology, University of Gothenburg.

—— 1995. 'The substance of kinship and the heat of the hearth: feeding, personhood, and relatedness among Malays in Pulau Langkawi', *American Ethnologist* 22, 223–41.

DepDikBud. 1992nd. *Sejarah Kecamatan Tombasian*, unpublished manuscript in Departemen Pendidikan dan Kebudayaan, Propinsi Sulawesi Utara, Kabupaten Minahasa, Kantor Kecamatan Tombasian.

Dube, L. 1986. 'Seed and earth: the symbolism of biological reproduction and sexual relations of production', in L. Dube, E. Leacock and S. Ardener, eds, *Visibility and Power. Essays on Women in Society and Development* Delhi, Oxford University Press.

Errington, S. 1983. 'Embodied sumange' in Luwu', *Journal of Asian Studies* 42, 45–70.

—— 1989. *Meaning and Power in a Southeast Asian Realm*, Princeton, N.J., Princeton University Press.

Firth, Raymond. [1946] 1966. *Malay Fishermen: Their Peasant Economy*, second edition, London, Routledge & Kegan Paul.

Firth, Rosemary. [1943] 1966. *Housekeeping among Malay Peasants*, London, Athlone Press.

Gandhi-Lapian, L. 1995. 'Persistence of adat law in Minahasa in the interests of justice, harmony and peace: aspects of family law for Christians in Minahasa', in R. Schefold, ed., *Minahasa Past and Present. Tradition and Transition in an Outer Island Region of Indonesia*, Leiden, Research School CNWS.

Graafland, N. [1869] 1991. *Minahasa. Negeri, Rakyat, dan Bidayanya*, trans. Lucy R. Montolalu, Jakarta, Yayasan Parahita.

Henley, D. [1992] 1995. *Nationalism and Regionalism in a Colonial*

Context. Minahasa in the Dutch East Indies, Leiden, KITLV Press.
Hickson, S.J. 1889. *A Naturalist in Northern Celebes. A narrative of travels in Minahassa, the Sangir and Talaut Island, with notices of the fauna, flora and ethnology of the districts visited*, London, John Murray.
Jones, G. W. 1977. *The Population of North Sulawesi*, ANU Indenosian Population Monograph Series, Yogyakarta, Gadjah Mada University Press.
Karsten, J. 1935. 'Primitive conception of the soul', in *The Origins of Religion*, London, Kegan Paul, Trenek, Trubier & Co.
Kotilainen, E.-M. 1992. '*When the Bones Are left*'. *A Study of the Material Culture of Central Sulawesi*, Helsinki, Transactions of the Finnish Anthropological Society no 3.
Kristanto, B. 1995. 'Sejarah masyaralat Borgo Tanawangko, Minahasa 191–1945, unpublished MSc thesis, Faculty of Letters, Sam Ratulangi University, Manado.
Kroeskamp, J. 1974. *Early Schoolmasters in a Developing Country*, Assen, Van Gorcum & Co.
Laderman, C. 1987. 'Destructive heat and cooling prayer: Malay humoralism in pregnancy, childbirth and the post-partum period', *Social Science and Medicine*, 25, 357–65.
—— 1991. *Taming the Wind of Desire. Psychology, Medicine, and Aesthetics in Malay Shamanistic Performance*, Berkeley, University of California Press.
Lundström, W. 1976. *The Group of People who Live in a House*, Working papers of the Department of Social Anthropology, University of Gothenburg.
Lundström-Burghoorn, W. 1981. *Minahasa Civilization. A Tradition of Change*, Gothenburg, Gothenburg Studies in Social Anthropology no 2.
van Olpen, A.J. 1843. 'Diverse Stukken over Manado (en Gorontalo'. First part of an unbound 377 folio manuscript. Archives of the Royal Institute of Linguistics and Anthropology, Leiden.
Sarwano, S. 1996. 'Personalistic belief in health. A case in West Java', in P. Boomgaard, R. Sciortino and I. Smyth, eds, Health Care in Java. Past and Present, Leiden, KITLV Press.
Schefold, R. 1995. 'Function follows form: on the ritual efficacy of plants and textiles in Indonesia', *Indonesia Circle* 66, 79–99.

Schouten, M. 1993. *Minahasan Metamorphoses. Leadership and Social Mobility in a Southeast Asian Society, c. 1680–1983.* Covilhã, Serviços Gráficos da Universidade da Beira Interior.

—— 1995. 'From *anak piara* to *PKK*: ideologies and history of Minahasan women's household duties'. A paper for the 3rd WIVS Conference on Indonesian Women's Studies & International Workshop on Indonesian Studies no 10. Leiden, 25–29 September 1995.

Schrauwers, A. 1995. 'The household and shared poverty in the highlands of Central Sulawesi, *Journal of the Royal Anthropological Institute* (N.S.) 1, 227–53.

Slamet-Velsink, I.E. 1996. 'Some reflections on the sense and nonsense of traditional health care', in P. Boomgaard, R. Sciortino and I. Smyth, eds, *Health Care in Java. Past and Present*, Leiden, KITLV Press.

Southon, M. 1995. *The Navel of the Perahu: Meaning and Values in the Maritime Trading Economy of a Butonese Village*, Canberra, Department of Anthropology, RSPacS, ANU.

TAD. 1987. *Pedoman untuk memanfaatkan Apotik Hidup*, Samarinda, TAD Subproject Health and Nutrition.

Volkman, T.A. 1985. *Feasts of Honour: Ritual and Change in the Toraja Higlands*. Urbana and Chicago, University of Illinois Press.

Wall, L.L. 1995. 'The anthropologist as obstetrician. Childbirth observed and childbirth experienced', *Anthropology Today* 11, 12–15.

Watuseke, F.S. 1968. *Sedjarah Minahasa*, Manado, Percetakan Negara.

Watuseke, F.S. and Henley, D.E.F. 1994. 'C.C. Predigers Verhandeling over het Plaatselijke Bestuur en de Huishouding van de Minahasa in 1804', *Bijdragen tot de Taal-, Land- en Volkenkunde* 150, 357–85.

Wikan, U. 1990. *Managing Turbulent Hearts. A Balinese Formula for Living*. Chicago, University of Chicago Press.

Wilken, G.A. 1921. *The Sociology of Malayan Peoples. Being Three Essays on Kinship, Marriage, and Inheritance on Indonesia*. Kuala Lumpur, Committee for Malay Studies.

Wilken, N.P. 1849. 'De godsdienst en godsdienstplegtigheden der Alfoeren in de Menahassa op het eiland Celebes', *Tijdschrift voor Nederlandsch-Indië* 11, 387–402.

CHAPTER 6

Baldick, J. 1993. *Imaginary Muslims. The Uwaysi Sufis of Central Asia*, London and New York, I.B. Tauris.

Bellér-Hann, I. 1995. 'Myth and history on the eastern Black Sea coast', *Central Asian Survey*, 14 (4), 487–508.

—— 1997. 'The peasant condition in Xinjiang', *The Journal of Peasant Studies*, 25 (1), 87–112.

Benninghaus, R. 1989. 'The Laz: an example of multiple identification', in P.A. Andrews, ed., *Ethnic Groups in the Republic of Turkey*, Wiesbaden, Otto Harrassowitz, 497–502.

Benson, Linda. 1993a. 'The Turkic peoples of China', in M. Bainbridge, ed., *The Turkic Peoples of the World*, London, Kegan Paul, 53–83.

—— 1993b. 'A much-married woman: marriage and divorce in Xinjiang 1850–1950', *Muslim World* 83 (3–4), 227–47.

Boserup, Ester. 1970. *Woman's Role in Economic Development*, New York, St Martin's Press.

Croll, Elizabeth. 1979. *Women in Rural Development. The People's Republic of China*, Geneva, International Labour Office.

Davin, Delia. 1976. *Woman-Work. Women and the Party in Revolutionary China*, Oxford, Clarendon Press.

Delaney, Carol. 1986. 'The meaning of paternity and the virgin birth debate', *Man* 21 (3), 494–513.

—— 1991. *The Seed and the Soil. Gender and Cosmology in Turkish Village Society*, Berkeley, University of California Press.

Dube, Leela. 1986. 'Seed and earth: the symbolism of biological reproduction and sexual relations of production', in L. Dube, E. Leacock and S. Ardener, eds, *Visibility and Power. Essays on Women in Society and Development*, Delhi, Oxford University Press, 22–53.

Feurstein, W. 1983. 'Untersuchungen zur Materiellen Kultur der Lazen', unpublished dissertation, [Magisterarbeit], Freiburg, Albert-Ludwigs-Universitat).

—— 1984. *Lazuri Alfabe; lazca alfabe; entwurf eines lazischen alphabetes (Parpali 1)*, Gundelfingen, Lazebura.

—— 1992. *Lasen. In Die Völker der Erde. Kulturen und Nationalitaten von A-Z*, Gutersloh/München, Bertelsmann Lexicon Verlag.

Gladney, Dru. 1991. *Muslim Chinese. Ethnic Nationalism in the People's Republic*, Cambridge, Mass., Council on East Asia Studies, Harvard University.

—— 1992. 'Transnational Islam and Uighur national identity: Salman Rushdie, Sino-Muslim missile deals, and the Trans-Eurasian Railway', *Central Asian Survey* 11 (3). 1–18.

Goody, Jack. 1976. *Production and Reproduction*, Cambridge, Cambridge University Press.

Grenard, F. 1898. *Mission scientifique dans la Haute Asie 1890-1895,* Paris, Ernest Leroux.

Häbibulla, A. 1993. *Uygur etnografiyisi*, Ürümçi, injang Xälq Näriyati.

Hann, C.M. 1990. *Tea and the domestication of the Turkish State,* SOAS Modern Turkish Studies Programme Occasional Papers 1, Huntingdon, The Eothen Press.

—— 1997. 'Ethnicity, language and politics in north-east Turkey', in C. Govers and H. Vermeulen, eds, *The Politics of Ethnic Consciousness*, London, Macmillan, 121--56.

Jarring, G. 1946–51. *Materials to the Knowledge of Eastern Turki*, parts I–IV, Lund, The University of Lund.

—— 1992. 'Garments from top to toe. Eastern Turki texts relating to articles of clothing', edited with translation, notes and glossary. *Scripta Minora* 1991–2 (2), 1–93.

Jeffery, Roger and Jeffery, Patricia. 1993. 'Traditional birth attendants in rural north India. The social organization of childbearing', in S. Lindenbaum and M. Lock, eds., *Knowledge, Power and Practice. The Anthropology of Medicine and Everyday Life*, Berkeley, University of California Press, 7–31.

Katanov, N.T. and Menges K.H. [1933] 1976. 'Volkskundliche Texte aus Ost-Turkistan', Aus dem Nachlass von N. Th. Katanov herausgegeben von K. H. Menges ... in *Sitzungsberichte der preussischen*, Akademie der Wissenschaften Philologisch-Historische Klasse, 1933. Berlin, 1163–1293; reprinted 1976; Leipzig, Zentralantiquariat der Deutschen Demokratischen Republik.

Khatib-Chahidi, Jane. 1981. 'Sexual prohibitions, shared space and fictive marriages in Shi'ite Iran', in S. Ardener ed., *Women and Space. Ground Rules and Social Maps,* London, Croom Helm.

Lattimore, O. 1950. *Pivot of Asia*, Boston, Little, Brown.

MacCormack, C.P. 1982. 'Biological, cultural and social

adaptation in human fertility and birth: a synthesis', in C. MacCormack, ed., *Ethnography of Fertility and Birth*, London, Academic Press, 1–13.

Mackerras, Colin. 1995. *China's Minority Cultures: Identities and Integration Since 1912*, New York, St Martin's Press.

Marr, N. 1910. 'Iz poezdki v Tureckij Lazistan', *Bulletin de l'Academie Imperiale des Sciences de St.-Petersbourg*, 6th series, 547–632.

Meeker, Michael. 1970. 'The Black Sea Turks: a study of honor, descent and marriage', unpublished thesis, University of Chicago.

—— 1971. 'The Black Sea Turks: some aspects of their ethnic and cultural background', *International Journal of Middle Eastern Studies*, 2 (4), 318–345.

Millward, J.A. 1993. 'Beyond the Pass: Commerce, Ethnicity and the Qing Empire in Xinjiang, 1759–1864', unpublished PhD dissertation, University of Stanford.

Prov. 207.I-II. Unpublished manuscript, Lund University Library.

Prov. 212. Unpublished manuscript, Lund University Library.

Prov. 464. Unpublished manuscript, Lund University Library.

Raxman, A., Hämdulla, R. and . Xutar. 1996. *Uygur örp-adätliri.* [Uighur traditions]. Ürümçi, injang Yalar-Ösmürlär Näriyati.

Rize'de el Sanatlar. 1991. *Rize: Halk Egitim Müdürlügü.* Typescript.

Rudelson, Justin. 1997. *Oasis identities. Uyghur Nationalism along China's Silk Road*, New York, Columbia University Press.

Schwarz, Henry G. 1992. *An Uyghur–English Dictionary*, Washington, Western Washington University.

Searle, John R. 1979. 'Metaphor', in A. Ortony, ed., *Metaphor and Thought*, Cambridge, Cambridge University Press, 92–123.

Stirling, P. and E. Onaran Incirioğlu. 1996. 'Choosing spouses: villagers, migrants, kinship and time', in G. Rasuly-Paleczek, ed., *Turkish Families in Transition*, Frankfurt am Main, Peter Lang.

Tenishev, E.R. 1984. *Ujgurskie teksty*, Moscow, Nauka.

Toumarkine, A. 1991. *Les Lazes en Turquie (XIXe–XXe siecle)*, Istanbul, Isis.

Warikoo, K.B. 1985. 'Chinese Turkestan during the nineteenth century, a socio-economic study', *Central Asian Survey* 4 (3), 75–114.

CHAPTER 7

Abu-Lughod, L. 1993. 'Islam and the gendered discourses of wealth', *International Journal of Middle East Studies* 25, 187–205.

Al-Azhar. 1992). 'Ahkam el-Zawag we el-Ingab' (injunctions on marriage and reproduction, Al-Azhar Mosque, Cairo; Al-Azhar Press.

Ali, K. 1996. 'Notes on rethinking masculinities: an Egyptian case', in S. Zeidenstein and Kirsten Moore, eds, *Learning About Sexuality: A Practical Beginning*, New York, The Population Council, 98–110.

Appadurai, Arjun. 1988. 'Putting hierarchy in its place', *Cultural Anthropology* 3, 36–49.

Bouhdiba, A. 1985. *Sexuality in Islam*, trans. Alan Sheridan, London, Routledge and Kegan Paul.

Delaney, Carol. 1986. 'The meaning of paternity and the virgin birth debate', *Man* 21 (3), 494–513.

—— 1991. *The Seed and the Soil: Gender and Cosmology in Turkish Village Society*, Berkeley, University of California Press.

El-Ghazaly, M. 1990. 'Hiya' 'Oulum ed Deen (in Arabic) (*The Reincarnation/Renaissance of Religious Learning*) Cairo; Photocopy.

Inhorn, M. 1994. *Quest for Conception: Gender Infertiliity and Egyptian Medical Traditions*, Philadelphia, University of Pennsylvania Press.

IRRRAG. 1996. 'Women's Reproductive Rights in Egypt', in *International Reproductive Rights Research and Action Group Report*, unpublished.

Mernissi, F. 1987. *Beyond the Veil: Male Female Dynamics in Modern Muslim Society*, Bloomington, Indiana University Press.

—— 1991. *Women and Islam: An Historical and Theological Inquiry*, trans. Mary Jo Lakeland, Oxford, Basil Blackwell.

Mir-Hosseini, Z. 1994. *Marriage on Trial*, Cambridge, Cambridge University Press.

Morsy, S. 1988. 'Islamic Clinics in Egypt: the cultural elaboration of biomedical hegemony', *Medical Anthropology Quarterly* 2 (4), 355–369.

Raggab, A., Serrour, G., et al. 1996. 'The position of Muslim culture towards abortion', *Population Sciences: International Islamic Center for Population Studies and Research*, Al Azhar University, 16, (July), 1–18.

Sabbah, F. 1984. *Women in the Muslim Unconscious*, The Athene Series, New York, Pergamon Press.

CHAPTER 8

Bloch, M. 1975. 'Property and the end of affinity', in M. Bloch, ed., *Marxist Analyses and Social Anthropology*, London, Malaby Press, 203–22.

—— 1992. 'What goes without saying: the conceptualization of Zafimaniry society', in A Kuper, ed., *Conceptualising Society*, London, Routledge, 127–46.

Bloch, M. and Parry, J. eds. 1982. *Death and the Regeneration of Life,* Cambridge, Cambridge University Press.

Christian, W. 1989. *Person and God in a Spanish Valley*, Princeton, Princeton University Press.

Davis, J. 1984. 'The sexual division of religious labour in the Mediterranean', in E.R. Wolf, ed., *Religion, Power, and Protest in Local Communities,* Berlin, Mouton, 17–50.

Delaney, C. 1986. 'The meaning of paternity and the Virgin Birth debate'. *Man* 21, 494–513.

—— 1991. *The Seed and the Soil: Gender and Cosmology in Turkish Village Society,* Berkeley, University of California Press.

Dube, L. 1986. *Visibility and Power: Essays on Women in Society and Development,* Delhi, Oxford University Press.

du Boulay, J. 1991. 'Cosmos and gender in village Greece', in P. Loizos and E. Paptaxiarchis, eds, *Contested Identities: Gender and Kinship in Modern Greece,* New Jersey, Princeton University Press, 47–78.

Goody, J. 1976. *Production and Reproduction: A Comparative Study of the Domestic Domain*, Cambridge, Cambridge University Press.

Gortani, L. [1898] 1981.'Usi, costumi, leggende e tradizioni', in G. Marinelli, ed., *Guida della Carnia*, Udine, Del Bianco.

Heady, P. 1999. *The Hard People: Rivalry, Sympathy and Social Structure in an Alpine Valley*, Chur, Switzerland, Harwood Academic.

Pina-Cabral, J. de. 1986. *Sons of Adam, Daughters of Eve*, Oxford, Clarendon Press.

Verdier, Y. 1990. 'Les femmes et le saloir. Le langage du cochon', in T. Jolas, M.-C. Pingaud, Y. Verdier and F. Zonabend, eds, *Une Campagne Voisine*, Paris, Editions de la maison des sciences de l'homme.

CHAPTER 9

du Boulay, J. 1986. 'Women – images of their nature and destiny in rural Greece', in J. Dubisch, *Gender and Power in Rural Greece*, Princeton, Princeton University Press, 139–168.

Rheubottom, D. 1976. 'The saint's feast and Skopska Crna Gora social structure', *Man* 11, 181–34.

—— 1980. 'Dowry and wedding celebrations in Yugoslav Macedonia', in J. Comaroff, ed., *The Meaning of Marriage Payments*, London, Academic Press.

—— 1993. 'The seed of evolution', in D. Parkin, ed., *The Anthropology of Evil*, Oxford, Blackwell.

Todorova, M.N. 1993. *Balkan Family Structure and the European Pattern: Demographic Developments in Ottoman Bulgaria*, Washington, D.C.;The American University Press.

CHAPTER 10

*Denotes the titles of Greek works that have been translated.

Abbott, G.F. 1903. *Macedonian Folklore*, Cambridge, Cambridge University Press.Agapios. 1850. *Agricultural Almanac*, Venice.*

Argenti, P. and Rose, H. 1949. *The Folklore of Chios*, 2 vols, Cambridge, Cambridge University Press.

Athanassopoulos, T. 1915. 'Magical rites for bearing children', *Laografia* 3, 408–9.*

Bloch, M. and Guggenheim, S. 1981. 'Compadrazgo, baptism and the symbolism of a second birth', *Man* 16(3), 376–86.

Bloch, M. and Parry, J. 1982. *Death and the Regeneration of Life*, Cambridge, Cambridge University Press.

Blum, R. and Blum, E. 1965. *Health and Healing in Rural Greece*, Stanford, Stanford University Press.

—— 1970. *The Dangerous Hour*, London, Chatto and Windus.

Bourdieu, Piere. 1970. 'La maison Kabyle ou le Monde Renversé', in *Echanges et Communications, Mélanges Offerts à*

C.Lévi-Strauss à l' Occasion de son 60e Anniversaire, Paris-La Haye, Mouton.

Boutouras, A. 1931. *Superstitions of the Greek People and their Interpretations*, Athens.

Brandes, S. 1981. 'Like wounded stages: male sexual ideology in an Andalusian town', in S. Ortner and H. Whitehead, eds, *Sexual Meanings*, Cambridge, Cambridge University Press, 216–239.

Brandstrom, P. 1990. 'Seeds and soil: the quest for life and the domestication of fertility in Sukuma-Nyamwezi thought and reality', in A. Jacobson-Widding and W. van Beek, eds, *The Creative Communion*, Uppsala, Almqvist and Wiksell International.

Brown, R.H. 1977. *A Poetic for Sociology*, Chicago and London, Chicago University Press.

Buckley, T. and Gottlieb, A. 1988. *Blood Magic: The Anthropology of Menstruation,* Berkeley, University of California Press.

Campbell, J. 1964. *Honour, Family and Patronage*, Oxford, Clarendon Press.

Chourmouziadis, C. 1940. 'The child in the ecclesiastical region of Athyras and Metrai in eastern Trace', *Archion Thrakicou Laograficou kai Glossikou Thessavrou* 7.*

Danforth, L. 1989. *Firewalking and Religious Healing*, Princeton, Princeton University Press.

Delaney, C. 1986. 'The meaning of paternity and the virgin birth debate', *Man* 21(3), 494–513.

—— 1991. *The Seed and the Soil*, Berkeley, University of California Press.

Dimitriou, N. 1983. *Folklore of Samos*, I, Athens.*

Douglas, M. 1966. *Purity and Danger*, London, Routledge and Kegan Paul.

Dube, L. 1986. 'Seed and earth: the symbolism of biological reproduction and sexual relations of production', in L. Dube, E. Leacock and S. Ardener, eds, *Visibility and Power*, Delhi, Oxford University Press, 22–53.

du Boulay, J. 1974. *Portrait of a Greek Mountain Village*, Oxford, Clarendon Press.

—— 1991. 'Cosmos and gender in village Greece', in P. Loizos and E. Papataxiarchis, eds, *Contested Identities*, Princeton, Princeton University Press.

Du Bois, P. 1988. *Sowing the Body*, Chicago and London, Cambridge University Press.

Frangaki, E. 1969. *A Contribution to the Folk Terminology of Plants*, Athens.*

—— 1974. *The Folk Art of Crete III: Weaving and Dyeing, Athens.**

—— 1978. *The Folk Medicine of Crete*, Athens.*

Gélis, J. 1984. *L' Arbre et le Fruit*, Paris, Fayard.

Handman, M.-E. 1980. 'La Vie d' une Communauté Villagoise: Domination Masculine et Violence à Pouri', Ph.D. dissertation, University of Paris X, Nanterre.

Heritier-Augé, F. 1985. 'Le Sperme et le Sang', *Nouvelle Revue de Psychanalyse* 32.

Herzfeld, M. 1982. *Ours Once More: Folklore, Ideology and the Making of Modern Greece,* Austin, University of Texas Press.

Holland D. and N. Quinn, eds. 1987. *Cultural Models in Language and Thought*, Cambridge, Cambridge University Press.

ILLA, *Historical Lexicon of the Athens Academy*, Athens.*

Kalyvi, K. 1938, *The Folklore of Cymi in Eubea*, Athens.*

Karapatakis, C. 1979. *Mother and Child in Older Times*, Athens.*

Keramida, O. 1932. 'Customs, beliefs, and superstitions from Stromnitsa concerning the child', *Laografia* 10, 449–58.*

Khaviara-Karachaliou, S. 1993. *The Folk Medicine of Chios*, Athens, Gasci-Hellas.*

Konsolas, N. 1966. 'Folklore from Olympos of Karpathos', *Laografia* 24.*

Koukoules, F. 1957. *Byzantine Life and Culture*, VI, Athens, The Athens French Institute.*

Kouzis, A. n.d. 'Folk medicine', in *Megali Elliniki Engyclopedia*, Athens.*

Kriaris, A. 1909. *Cretan Songs*, Khania.*

Kritopoulos, T. 1893. 'Confession of faith', in I. Messoloras, ed., *The Symbolic Books of Orthodox Eastern Church,* Athens.*

Kyriakidis, S. 1922. *Greek Folklore*, I. Athens.*

Kyriakidou-Nestoros, A. 1975. *Folklore Studies*, Athens, Olkos.*

Lakoff G. and Johnson, M. 1980. *Metaphors We Live By*, Chicago, Chicago University Press.

Lambrakis, C. 1915. 'Songs of Tsoumerca', *Laografia* 5.*

Laqueur, T. 1990. *Making Sex*, Cambridge, Mass., Harvard University Press.

Loizos, P. and Papataxiarchis, E., eds. 1991. *Contested Identities:* Princeton, Princeton University Press.

Loukatos, D. 1957. *Greek Folkloric Texts*, Athens, Zacharopoulos.*

Loukopoulos, D. 1938. *Agricultural Life and Customs of Roumeli*, Athens.*

Lyberis, N. 1975. *Folklore Material from Ambelos of Patras*, Patras.*

MacCormack, E.R. 1990. *A Cognitive Theory of Metaphor,* Cambridge Mass., and London, The MIT Press.

McGilvray, D.B. 1982. 'Sexual power, and fertility in Sri Lanka: Batticaloa Tamils and Moors', in C. MacCormack, ed., *Ethnography of Fertility and Birth,* New York, Academic Press. 15–64.

Marinellis, E. 1978. 'Birth, marriage, and death in Souli of Patras', *Laografia* 31.*

Megas, G. 1929. 'Adam and Christ in the traditions of the people', *Imerologio tis Megalis Ellados.**

—— 1939. *Questions of Greek Folklore*, part A, Athens, Epetiris Laograficou Archiou Acadimias Athinon.*

—— 1941–2, *Questions of Greek Folklore*, parts B and C, Athens, Epetiris Laograficou Archiou Acadimias Athinon.*

—— 1956, *Greek Calendar Customs*, Athens.*

Michailides-Nouaros, M. [1932] 1969. *Folkloric Miscellanea of Karpathos*, I, Athens.*

MLEG. 1964, *Mega Lexicon tis Ellinikis Glossis*, Athens, Dimitrakos.*

Musallam, B.F. 1983. *Sex and Society in Islam*, Cambridge, Cambridge University Press.

Onians, R.B. 1951. *The Origin of European Thought*, Cambridge, Cambridge University Press.

Opie, I. and Tatem, M., eds. 1989. *A Dictionary of Superstitions*, Oxford, Oxford University Press.

Overing, J. 1991. 'Today I shall call him mummy: multiple worlds and classificatory confusion', in J. Overing, ed., *Reason and Morality*, London and New York,Tavistock Publications, 152–79.

Papamichael, E. 1910. 'The wedding in Vourvoura of Kynouria', *Laografia* 2, 399–404.*

Papathanassi-Moussiopoulou, K. 1979. *The Folklore of Thrace*, I, Athens.*

—— 1981. *Folk Metaphysics*, Athens.*

Papazaphiropoulos, P. 1887. *Compilation of Linguistic Material and Customs of the Greek People*, Patras.*

Parkin, D. 1987. 'Comparison as the search for continuity', in L. Holy, ed., *Comparative Anthropology*, Oxford, Blackwell, 52–69.
Pedalion. [1800] 1976. *Canon Law of the Orthodox Church*, edited by Agapios and Nicodemus of the Holy Mountain, Athens, Astir.*
Petropoulos, D. 1954. *La Comparaison dans la Chanson Populaire Grecque,* Athens, Athens French Institute.
Pina-Cabral, J. de 1986. *Sons of Adam, Daughters of Eve*, Oxford,Clarendon Press.
Politis, N. 1874. *Modern Greek Mythology*, Athens.*
—— 1899–1902, *Studies of the Life and Language of the Greek People: Proverbs*, 4, Athens.*
—— 1904. *Studies of the Life and Language of the Greek People: Traditions*, 2, Athens.*
—— 1914. *Selections from the Songs of the Greek People*, Athens, Estia.*
—— [1921] 1975. *Folkloric Miscellanea*, II, Athens*
—— 1931. *Papers on Folklore*, 3, Athens,Athens Academy.*
Psychogios, N. 1951. 'Childrearing in Elia', *Laografia* 13, 340–6.*
—— 1989. *On Spells and Divination*, Lechena.*
Pyrros, D. 1831. *A Doctor's M*anual, 2 vols, Naplion.
Regas, A. 1970. *The Folk Culture of Skiathos*, 4, Salonica.*
Rodd, R. 1892. *The Customs and Lore of Modern Greece*, London, D. Scott.
Romaios, C. 1923. 'The use of ploughshare in weddings', *Laografia* 7, 346–68.*
Salmond, A. 1982. 'The theoretical landscapes: on cross-cultural conceptions of knowledge', in D. Parkin, ed., *Semantic Anthropology*, London, Academic Press, 65–87.
Salvanos, G. 1929. 'Miscellaneous Folkloric Material from Argyrades of Corfu', *Laografia* 10.*
Sanders, I.T. 1962. *Rainbow in the Rock: The People of Rural Greece*, Cambridge, Mass., Harvard University Press.
Sapir D. and J. Cristopher Crocker, eds. 1977. *The Social Use of Metaphor,* Philadelphia, University of Pennsylvania Press.
Saranti-Stamouli, E. 1933. 'Customs of Trace', *Thracica* 4, 312–43.
—— 1937. 'How they used to cure people in Thrace, A', *Thracica* 8, 350–83.*
—— 1938a. 'How they used to cure people in Thrace, B', *Thracica* 9, 195–283.*

—— 1952. 'Superstitions of Thrace', *Laografia* 14, 169–200.*
Searle, J. 1979. 'Metaphor', in A. Ortony, ed., *Metaphor and Thought*, Cambridge, Cambridge University Press.
Servier, J. 1985. *L' Homme et lM Invisible*, Paris, Rocher.
Sternberg, R.J. 1990. *Metaphors of Mind*, Cambridge, Cambridge University Press.
Stewart, C. 1991. *Demons and the Devil*, Princeton, Princeton University Press.
Theros, A. 1951. *Songs of the Greeks*, I, Athens, Zakharopoulos.*
Tsitselis, E. 1874. 'A glossary of the dialect of Cephalonia', *Neoellinica Analecta Parnassou*, II.*
Vanazounta, M. 1963. 'Questions concerning the child in Salamis', *Laografia* 21.*
Unpublished manuscripts of the Center for Research on Greek Folklore, Athens.
KL 1405, material collected by C. Bentas, 3/2/1939. Informant: E. Papountza (73 years old), Siatista, Macedonia.
KL 1566, coll. M. Tsakona, 1944. Inf.: Katsoulena (80 years old), Maniaki, Peloponnese.
KL 1628, coll. M. Kokkinis, 1950. Inf.: P. Spyratou (70 years old), Patras.
KL 1631, coll. P. Frangelis, 1950. Inf.: no names are given, Lesbos Island.
KL 1653, coll. D. Moussouri, 1950 (the material refers to 1870). Inf.: no names are given, villages of Attica region.
KL 1675, D. Pantazis, n.d. Inf.: no names are given, Mazi and Evangelistsra, Boetia.
KL 1953, coll. L. Simos, 1953. Inf.: no names are given, Amorgos Island, Cyclades.
KL 2125, coll. S. Karambelas, 1954. Inf.: no names are given, Skillountia, Olympia.
KL 2143, coll. P. Michelis, n.d. Inf.: no names are given, Limnos Island.

CHAPTER II

Ackrill, J.R. ed. 1987 *A New Aristotle Reader*, Oxford, Oxford University Press.
Aeschylus. 1953. *Oresteia,* trans. Richard Lattimore, Chicago, University of Chicago Press.
—— 1975. *The Oresteia*, trans. Robert Fagels, New York, Viking Press.

Allen, Garland. 1978. *Life Science in the Twentieth Century*, Cambridge, Cambridge University Press.

Aristotle. 1968. *Poetics*, trans. With an introduction by Malcolm Heath, London, Penguin.

—— 1984.'The generation of animals', trans. A Platt, in J. Barnes, ed., *The Complete Works of Aristotle*, vol 8, Princeton, Princeton University Press.

Astruc, J. 1762. *A Treatise on the Diseases of Women*, London, J. Nourse Bookseller.

Atkinson, Clarissa W. 1991. *The Oldest Vocation*, Christian Motherhood in the Middle Ages, Ithaca, Cornell University Press.

Baer, Karl Ernst von, 1827. *De Ovi Mammalium et Hominis Genesi Epistola*, Leipzig, L. Voss.

—— 1956. 'On the genesis of the ovum of mammals and of man', trans. Charles Donald O'Malley, introduction by I. Bernard Cohen, *ISIS*, 47, 117(Transl. Charles Donald O'Malley), 53.

—— 1986 (first edition 1886). *Autobiography of Dr Karl Ernst von Baer*, ed. Jane M. Oppenheimer, Canton, Mass., Watson Publishing International.

Barlow, Nora. 1958. *The Autobiography of Charles Darwin, 1809–1882*, London, Collins.

Bodemer, Charles W. 1964. 'Regeneration and the decline of preformationism in eighteenth century embryology', *Bulletin of the History of Medicine*, 28, 20–31.

—— 1968. 'Embryological thought in seventeenth century England', in *Medical Investigations in Seventeenth Century England,* Los Angeles, University of California,William Andrews Clark Memorial Library.

Bord, Janet and Colin. 1982. 'Fertility practices in pre-industrial Britain', in *Earth Rites*, London, Granada.

Bouhdiba, Abdelwahab. 1985. *Sexuality in Islam*, trans. Alan Sheridan, London, Routledge and Kegan Paul.

Bowler, Peter J, 1971. 'Preformation and Pre-existence in the Seventeenth Century, A Brief Analysis', *Journal of the History of Biology*, Vol. 4, No.2. (Fall), pp. 221-244.

—— 1973. 'Bonnet and Buffron: theories of generation and the problem of species', *Journal of the History of Biology*, 6, (2), (Fall), 259–81.

—— 1975. 'The changing meaning of evolution', *Journal of the History of Ideas*, 36, pp. 95–114.

—— 1989. 'Darwin on man in the Origin of Species: a reply to Carl Bajema', *Journal of the History of Biology*, 22, (3), (Fall), 497–500.

Boylan, Michael. 1984. 'The Galenic and Hippocratic challenges to Aristotle's conception theory', *Journal of the History of Biology*, 17 (1) (Spring), 83–112.

Brooks, William Keith. 1883. *The Law of Heredity*, Baltimore, John Murphy.

Churchill, Frederick B. 1968. 'August Weisman and a break from tradition', *Journal of the History of Biology*, 1 (1) (Spring), 91–112.

—— 1970. 'Hertwig, Weismann and the meaning of reduction division', *ISIS* 61, 429–57.

—— 1970. 'The history of embryology as intellectual history', *Journal of the History of Biology*, 3 (1) (Spring), 155–81.

—— 1973. 'Sex and the single organism: biological theories of sexuality in the mid nineteenth century', *Studies in the History of Biology* 3, 139–77.

—— 1987. 'From heredity theory to Vererbung', *ISIS* 78, 337–64.

Cole, F.J. 1930. *Early Theories of Sexual Generation*, Oxford, Clarendon Press.

Coleman, William. 1965. 'Cell, nucleus and inheritance: an historical study', *Proceedings of the American Philosophical Society* 109, 124–58.

Cooke, J. 1762. *The New Theory of Reproduction*, London, J Buckland.

Croft, L.R., 1989. *The Life and Death of Charles Darwin*, Chorley, Elmwood.

Cronin, H. 1991. *The Ant and the Peacock: Altruism and Sexual Selection from Darwin to Today*, Cambridge, Cambridge University Press.

Darlington, C.D. 1964. *Genetics and Man*, London, George Allen and Unwin.

Darwin, Charles. 1859. *On the Origin of Species*, London, Murray.

Darwin, Erasmus. 1794. Zoomania: Or the Laws of Organic Life, vol. I, London, Walter Scott.

Delaney, Carol. 1991. *The Seed and the Soil*, Berkeley, University of California Press.

Dobell, Clifford. 1960 *Antony von Leeuwenhoek and His Little Animals*, New York, Dover.

Farley, John. 1977. *Ideas about Sexual Reproduction 1750–1914: Gametes and Spores* Baltimore and London, The Johns Hopkins University Press.

Foote, Edward T. 1969. 'Harvey: spontaneous generation and the egg', *Annals of Science*, 25, 139–63.

Frazer, J.G. [1890]1980. *The Golden Bough: A Study in Magic and Religion*, London, Papermac.

Galen, 1968 *On the Usefulness of the Parts of the Body*, trans. M. May, Ithaca, Cornell University Press.

Garden, George. 1691. 'A discourse concerning the modern theory of generation', *Philosophical Transactions of the Royal Society*, 17, 474–83.

Gasking, Elizabeth R. 1967. *Investigations into Generation 1651–1828*, London, Hutchinson.

Geddes, Patrick. 1889. *The Evolution of Sex*, London, Walter Scott.

Ginzberg, Louis. 1956. *Legends of the Bible*, Philadelphia, The Jewish Publication Society of America.

Glass, Bentley. 1959. 'Maupertuis, pioneer of genetics and evolution', in B. Glass et al., eds, *Forerunners of Darwin: 1745–1859,* Baltimore, Johns Hopkins University Press.

Goode, John Mason. 1813. Pantologia, A New Cyclopaedia, London, Kearsley.

—— 1826. *The Book of Nature.*

Graham, Harvey. 1950. *Eternal Eve*, London, William Heinemann.

Haeckel, Ernst. 1993. *The Riddle of the Universe (At the Close of the Nineteenth Century), 1899*, trans. by Joseph McCabe, Buffalo, N.Y., Prometheus Books.

Harding, Sandra. 1991. *Whose Science? Whose Knowledge*?, Milton Kynes, Open University Press.

Harvey, William, n.d. *Disputations Touching the Generation of Animals,* Oxford, Blackwell Scientific Publications.

Hewson, M. Anthony. 1975. *Giles of Rome and the Medieval Theory of Conception,* London, Athlone.

Hertwig, Oscar. 1896. *The Biological Problem of To-day: Preformation or Epigenesis? The Basis of a Theory of Organic Development*, trans. P. Chalmers Mitchell, London, W. Heinemann.

Hertig, Arthur T. 1989. 'A fifteen-year search for first-stage human ova', *The Journal of the American Medical Association*, 261, (3) (20 Jan), 434–5.

Holmes, S.J. 1947. 'K.E. Von Baer's perplexities over Evolution', *ISIS* 37, 7–14.

Horowitz, Maryanne Cline. 1976. 'Aristotle and women', *Journal of the History of Biology* 9 (2), (Fall), 183–213.

Hubbard, Ruth. 1990. *The Politics of Women's Biology*, New Brunswick, Rutgers Press.

Jacob, François. 1973. *The Logic of Life: A History of Heredity*, trans. Betty E. Spillmann, London, Allen Lane.

Kennon, Donald R. 1984. 'An apple of discord: the woman question at the world's anti-slavery convention of 1840', *Slavery & Abolition* 5 (3) (December).

Laqueur, Thomas. 1990. *Making Sex: Body and Gender from the Greeks to Freud*, Cambridge Mass., Harvard University Press.

Leeuwenhoek, Antony Van. 1685. *Philosophical Transactions of the Royal Society* 25, 1120–34.

Longo, Frank J. 1987. *Fertilisation*, London, Chapman and Hall.

Lowndes Sevely, Josephine. 1987. *Eve's Secrets*, London, Bloomsbury.

Maupertuis, P.L.M. 1745. Venus Physique. Leyde. Repr. 1966.

McLaren, Angus. 1984. Reproductive Rituals: *The Perception of Fertility in England from the Sixteenth Century to the Nineteenth Century*, London, Methuen.

Meyer, William Arthur. 1938. 'A summary of von Baer's commentary', *Bulletin of the Institute of the History of Medicine*, 6, 1031–40.

—— 1939. *The Rise of Embryology*, London, Oxford University Press.

—— 1956. *Human Generation; Conclusions of Burdach, Dollinger and von Baer,* Stanford, Calif., Stanford University Press.

Miles, Margaret R. 1992. *Carnal Knowing: Female Nakedness and Religious Meaning in the Christian West*, Tunbridge Wells, Burns and Oates.

Morsink, Johannes. 1979. 'Was Aristotle's biology sexist?' *Journal of the History of Biology*, 12 (1) (Spring), 82–112.

Needham, Joseph. 1934. *A History of Embryology*, Cambridge, Cambridge University Press.

O'Faolain, Julia and Martines, Lauro. 1973. *Not in God's Image*, London, Temple Smith.

Oppenheimer, Jane. 1963. 'K.E. von Baer's beginning insights into causal-analytical relationships during development', *Developmental Biology* 7, 11–21.

—— 1967. *Essays in the History of Embryology and Biology*, Cambridge, Mass., MIT Press.

Ospovat, Don. 1976. 'The influence of Karl Ernst von Baer's embryology, 1828-1859: a reappraisal in light of Richard Owen's and William B. Carpenter's "Palaeontological applications of Von Baer's Law"', *Journal of the History of Biology* 9 (1) (Spring), 1–28.

Payne, Alma Smith. 1970. *The Cleere Observer: A Biography of Antoni van Leeuwenhoek*, London, Macmillan.

Plato. 1982. *The Republic*, vol. V, trans. Paul Shorey, Cambridge, Mass., Harvard University Press.

Preus, Anthony. 1970. 'Science and philosophy in Aristotle's *Generation of Animals*', *Journal of the History of Biology*, 3 (1) (Spring), 1–52.

—— 1977. 'Galen's criticism of Aristotle's conception theory', *Journal of the History of Biology* 10 (1) (Spring), 65–85.

Price, Dorothy. 1967. *A Historical Review of Embryology and Intersexuality: Fact and Fancy*, Leiden, E.J. Brill.

Punnett, R.C. n.d. 'Ovists and animalculists', *American Naturalist* 62, 481–507.

Roe, Shirley A. 1979. 'Rationalism and Embryology: Caspar Friedrich Wolff's Theory of Epigenesis', *Journal of the History of Biology*, Vol. 12, No. 1. (Spring), pp.1-43.

—— 1981. *Matter, Life, and Generation: Eighteenth Century Embryology and the Haller-Wolff Debate*, Cambridge, Cambridge University Press.

Ruestow, Edward G. 1983. 'Images and ideas: Leeuwenhoek's perception of the spermatozoa', *Journal of the History of Biology* 16 (2) (Summer), 185–224.

Russett, Cynthia Eagle. 1989. *Sexual Science: The Victorian Construction of Womanhood,* Cambridge Mass., Harvard University Press.

Sarton, George. 1931. 'The discovery of the mammalian egg and the foundaton of modern embryology', *ISIS*, 16, 315–30.

Schullian, Dorothy M. 1976. 'Notes and events; two letters on epigenesis from John Turberville Needham to Albrecht von Haller', *Journal of the History of Medicine* January, 68–77.

Shettles, Lardrum. 1960. *Ovum Human*, published by the author.

Shorter, Edward. 1984. *A History of Women's Bodies,* Harmondsworth, Pelican.

Shuttle, Penelope and Redgrove, Peter. 1980. *The Wise Wound, Menstruation and Everywoman*, Harmondsworth, Penguin.

Smith, John Maynard. 1931. *Did Darwin get it Right?*, London, Penguin.

Thomson, Sir J. Arthur, and Geddes, Patrick. 1931. *Life; Outlines of General Biology*, New York, Harper & Brothers.

Tuana, Nancy. 1989a. 'The sexist bias of reproductive theory', in N. Tuana, ed., *Feminism and Society*, Bloomington, Indiana University Press.

—— 1989b. *Feminism and Science*, Bloomington, Indiana University Press.

Vetterling, Mary, Elliston, Frederick A., and English, Jane, eds, 1977. *Feminism and Philosophy*, Totowa, Littlefield Adams and Co.

Weigle, Marta. 1989. *Creation and Procreation*, Philadelphia, University of Pennsylvania Press.

Westermarck, Edward. 1921. *The History of Human Marriage*, London, Macmillan.

Zirkle, Conway. 1936. 'Animals impregnated by the wind', *ISIS* 25, 95–130.

Editors Note: Full references on many sources can be found in certain key works consulted by the author, e.g. Needham, J., Bodemer, C.W., Glass, B.

INDEX

LONDON SCHOOL OF ECONOMICS
MONOGRAPHS ON SOCIAL ANTHROPOLOGY

1 & 2 The Work of the Gods in Tikopia
RAYMOND FIRTH
0 485 19501 1 (2nd edn in one volume) hb

14 Chinese Spirit-Medium Cults in Singapore (Second Edition)
ALAN J. A. ELLIOTT
With a new Preface by Sir Raymond Firth
0 485 19514 3 hb

17 Indigenous Political Systems of Western Malaya
J. M. GULLICK
0 485 19417 1 Rev edn hb

19 Political Leadership among Swat Pathans
FREDRIK BARTH
0 485 19619 0 pb

20 Social Status and Power in Java
L. H. PALMIER
0 485 19620 4 pb

22 Rethinking Anthropology
E. R. LEACH
0 485 19622 0 pb

24 Legal Institutions in Manchu China
A Sociological Analysis
SYBILLE VAN DER SPRENKEL
0 485 19624 7 Revised edn pb

28 Essays on Social Organization and Values
RAYMOND FIRTH
0 485 19628 X pb

33 Chinese Lineage and Society
Fukien and Kwantung
MAURICE FREEDMAN
0 485 19633 6 pb

37 Kinship and Marriage among the Anlo Ewe
G. K. NUKUNYA
0 485 19637 9 pb

38 Anthropology and Social Change
LUCY MAIR
0 485 19638 7 pb

39 Take Out Hunger
Two Case Studies of Rural Development in Basutoland
SANDRA WALLMAN
0 485 19539 9 hb

40 Time and Social Structure and Other Essays
MEYER FORTES
0 485 19540 2 hb

41 Report on the Iban
DEREK FREEMAN
0 485 19541 0 hb

42 The Political Structure of the Chinese Community in Cambodia
W. E. WILLMOTT
0 485 19542 9 hb

44 Political Systems of Highland Burma
A Study of Kachin Social Structure
E. R. LEACH
0 485 19644 1 pb

45 Pioneers in the Tropics
The Political Organization of Japanese in an Immigrant Community in Brazil
PHILIP STANIFORD
0 485 19543 3 hb

47 West Indian Migration
The Montserrat Case
STUART B. PHILPOTT
0 485 19547 X hb

48 Land and Family in Pisticci
J. DAVIS
0 485 19548 8 hb

49 Beyond the Village
Local Politics in Madang, Papua New Guinea
LOUISE MORAUTA
0 485 19549 6 hb

51 Metamorphosis of the Cassowaries
Umeda Society, Language and Ritual
ALFRED GELL
0 485 19551 8 hb

52 Knowledge of Illness in a Sepik Society
A Study of the Gnau, New Guinea
GILBERT LEWIS
0 485 19552 6 hb

53 White Nile Arabs
Political Leadership and Economic Change
ABBAS AHMED MOHAMED
0 485 19553 4 hb

54 Ma'Betisék Concepts of Living Things
WAZIR-JAHAN KARIM
9 485 19554 2 hb

55 Forest Traders
A Socio-Economic Study of the Hill Pandaram
BRIAN MORRIS
0 485 19555 0 hb

56 Communications, Social Structure and Development in Rural Malaysia
A Study of Kampung Kuala Bera
WILLIAM D. WILDER
0 485 19556 9 hb

57 Sacrifice and Sharing in the Philippine Highlands
Religion and Society among the Buid of Mindoro
THOAMS P. GIBSON
0 485 19559 3 hb

**58 Ritual, History and Power: **
Selected Papers in Anthropology
MAURICE BLOCH
0 485 19658 1 pb

59 Gods on Earth
The Management of Religious Experience and Identity in a North Indian Pilgrimage Centre
PETER VAN DER VEER
0 485 19510 0 hb

60 The Social Practice of Symbolization:
An Anthropological Analysis
IVO STRECKER
0 485 19557 7 hb

61 Making Sense of Hierarchy: Cognition as Social Process in Fiji
CHRISTINA TOREN
Fijian hierarchy and its constitution in everyday ritual behaviour
0 485 19561 5 hb

62 The Power of Love
The Moral Use of Knowledge amongst the Amuesha of Central Peru
FERNANDO SANTOS-GRANERO
0 485 19562 3 hb

63 Society and Politics in India:
Essays in a Comparative Perspective
ANDRE BETEILE
0 485 19563 1 hb

64 The Harambee Movement in Kenya
Self-Help, Developmnet and Education among the Kamba of Kitui District
MARTIN J. D. HILL
0 485 19564 X hb

65 Hierarchy and Egalitarianism: Caste, Class and Power in Sinhalese Peasant Society
TAMARA GUNASEKERA
'fascinating' W W Reinhardt *Journal of Social and Behavioural Sciences*
0 485 19565 8 hb

66 Leadership and Change in the Western Pacific
Edited by RICHARD FEINBERG and KAREN ANN WATSON-GEGEO
Essays presented to Sir Raymond Firth on the occasion of his 90th Birthday.
0 485 19566 6 hb

67 The Art of Anthropology: Essays and Diagrams
ALFRED GELL
0 485 19567 4 hb
0 485 19660 3 pb

68 Conceiving Persons: Ethnographies of Procreation, Fertility and Growth
Edited by PETER LOIZOS and P. HEADY
0 485 19568 2 hb

69 Those who Play with Fire: Gender, Fertility and Transformation in East and Southern Africa
Edited by HENRIETTA L. MOORE, TODD SANDERS and BWIRE KAARE
0 485 19569 0 hb

70 Arguments with Ethnography: Comparative Approaches to History, Politics and Religion
IOAN M. LEWIS
0 485 19570 4 hb